James A. Chu, MD
Elizabeth S. Bowman, MD
Editors

Trauma and Sexuality: The Effects of Childhood Sexual, Physical, and Emotional Abuse on Sexual Identity and Behavior

Trauma and Sexuality: The Effects of Childhood Sexual, Physical, and Emotional Abuse on Sexual Identity and Behavior has been co-published simultaneously as *Journal of Trauma & Dissociation*, Volume 3, Number 4 2002.

Pre-publication REVIEWS, COMMENTARIES, EVALUATIONS . . .

"Sexuality is one of the major domains of human life affected by childhood trauma–and not only by sexual trauma, but by all types of maltreatment and neglect. While in recent years sexuality, including sexual identity, has shed its skin of taboo, and subsequently it has become more acceptable to discuss sexual trauma, it is most surprising that trauma's impact on sexuality and gender has received so little scientific attention. In this unique book some of those make this highly charged area the focus of their scientific and clinical work have brought together their most recent findings and insights. They write about the range of healthy expressions of sexuality and gender

More pre-publication
REVIEWS, COMMENTARIES, EVALUATIONS . . .

identity and the impact of sexual trauma and dissociation on these expression; the development of a variety of dissociative 'feminine' and 'masculine' personality styles in sexually abused girls and boys; the continuum of sexual behaviors engaged in by abused children; hyposexuality and hypersexuality secondary to childhood trauma and dissociation; the impact of traumatic experiences on risk-behavior among HIV-positive adults; and speculate about the high proportion of the same-sex orientation found among individuals with dissociative identity disorder or dissociative disorder not otherwise specified. The clinical implications of all these findings and ideas receive ample attention.

Readers of this book will become informed of the cutting edge of work in the field of sexuality as it relates to trauma, which will help their work with trauma survivors. But more broadly, they will also become much more comfortable and emphatic in discussing gender issues and much better equipped to help heterosexual, gay, lesbian, bisexual, or transgendered clients deal with sexual problems and develop sexual intimacy."

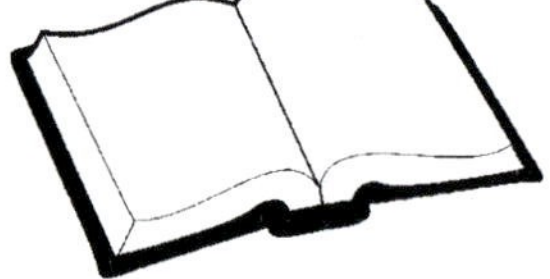

Onno van der Hart, PhD
Professor
Department of Clinical Psychology
Utrecht University
Utrecht, the Netherlands
President
International Society
for Traumatic Stress Studies

Trauma and Sexuality: The Effects of Childhood Sexual, Physical, and Emotional Abuse on Sexual Identity and Behavior

Trauma and Sexuality: The Effects of Childhood Sexual, Physical, and Emotional Abuse on Sexual Identity and Behavior has been co-published simultaneously as *Journal of Trauma & Dissociation*, Volume 3, Number 4 2002.

The *Journal of Trauma & Dissociation* Monographic "Separates"

Below is a list of "separates," which in serials librarianship means a special issue simultaneously published as a special journal issue or double-issue *and* as a "separate" hardbound monograph. (This is a format which we also call a "DocuSerial.")

"Separates" are published because specialized libraries or professionals may wish to purchase a specific thematic issue by itself in a format which can be separately cataloged and shelved, as opposed to purchasing the journal on an on-going basis. Faculty members may also more easily consider a "separate" for classroom adoption.

"Separates" are carefully classified separately with the major book jobbers so that the journal tie-in can be noted on new book order slips to avoid duplicate purchasing.

You may wish to visit Haworth's website at . . .

http://www.HaworthPress.com

. . . to search our online catalog for complete tables of contents of these separates and related publications.

You may also call 1-800-HAWORTH (outside US/Canada: 607-722-5857), or Fax 1-800-895-0582 (outside US/Canada: 607-771-0012), or e-mail at:

getinfo@haworthpressinc.com

Trauma and Sexuality: The Effects of Childhood Sexual, Physical, and Emotional Abuse on Sexual Identity and Behavior, edited by James A. Chu, MD, and Elizabeth S. Bowman, MD (Vol. 3, No. 4, 2002). *Examines the effects of childhood trauma on sexual orientation and behavior.*

Trauma and Sexuality: The Effects of Childhood Sexual, Physical, and Emotional Abuse on Sexual Identity and Behavior

James A. Chu, MD
Elizabeth S. Bowman, MD
Editors

Trauma and Sexuality: The Effects of Childhood Sexual, Physical, and Emotional Abuse on Sexual Identity and Behavior has been co-published simultaneously as *Journal of Trauma & Dissociation*, Volume 3, Number 4 2002.

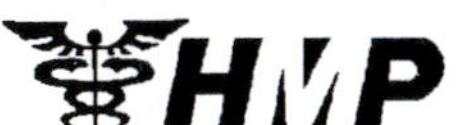

The Haworth Medical Press
The Haworth Maltreatment & Trauma Press
Imprints of
The Haworth Press, Inc.
New York • London • Oxford

Published by

The Haworth Medical Press®, 10 Alice Street, Binghamton, NY 13904-1580 USA

The Haworth Medical Press® is an imprint of The Haworth Press, Inc., 10 Alice Street, Binghamton, NY 13904-1580 USA.

Trauma and Sexuality: The Effects of Childhood Sexual, Physical, and Emotional Abuse on Sexual Identity and Behavior has been co-published simultaneously as *Journal of Trauma & Dissociation*, Volume 3, Number 4 2002.

Cover design by Marylouise E. Doyle

Library of Congress Cataloging-in-Publication Data

Trauma and sexuality : the effects of childhood sexual, physical, and emotional abuse on sexual identity and behavior / James A. Chu, Elizabeth S. Bowman, Editors.

p. cm.

Includes bibliographical references and index.

ISBN 0-7890-2042-4 (hard : alk. paper) – ISBN 0-7890-2043-2 (pbk. : alk. paper)

1. Adult child abuse victims–Sexual behavior. 2. Adult child abuse victims–Mental health. 3. Psychosexual disorders–Etiology. I. Chu, James A. II. Bowman, Elizabeth S.

RC569.5.C55 T735 2002

616.85′8369–dc21

2002015166

Indexing, Abstracting & Website/Internet Coverage

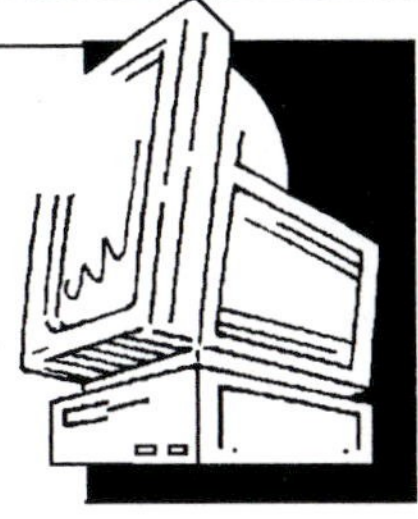

This section provides you with a list of major indexing & abstracting services. That is to say, each service began covering this periodical during the year noted in the right column. Most Websites which are listed below have indicated that they will either post, disseminate, compile, archive, cite or alert their own Website users with research-based content from this work. (This list is as current as the copyright date of this publication.)

Abstracting, Website/Indexing Coverage . . . . Year When Coverage Began

- ***Biology Digest (in print & online)*** **2000**
- ***CNPIEC Reference Guide: Chinese National Directory of Foreign Periodicals*** **2000**
- ***Contemporary Women's Issues*** **2000**
- ***EAP Abstracts Plus*** **2000**
- ***EMBASE/Excerpta Medica Secondary Publishing Division <www.elsevier.nl>*** **2000**
- ***e-psyche, LLC <www.e-psyche.net>*** **2001**
- ***Family & Society Studies Worldwide <www.nisc.com>*** **2000**
- ***Family Violence & Sexual Assault Bulletin*** **2000**
- ***FINDEX <www.publist.com>*** **2000**
- ***Gay & Lesbian Abstracts <www.nisc.com>*** **2000**
- ***IBZ International Bibliography of Periodical Literature <www.saur.de>*** **2001**
- ***Index to Periodical Articles Related to Law*** **2001**

(continued)

- ***Journal of Social Work Practice "Abstracts Section" <http://www.carfax.co.uk/jsw-ad.htm>*** **2000**
- ***MANTIS (Manual, Alternative and Natural Therapy) MANTIS is available through three database vendors: Ovid, Dialog & DataStar. In addition it is available for searching through <www.healthindex.com>*** **2000**
- ***National Clearinghouse on Child Abuse & Neglect Information Documents Database <www.calib.com/nccanch>*** **2000**
- ***PASCAL, c/o Institute de L'Information Scientifique et Technique <www.inst.fr>*** **2001**
- ***Psychiatric Rehabilitation Journal*** **2000**
- ***Psychological Abstracts (PsycINFO) <www.apa.org>*** **2001**
- ***Published International Literature on Traumatic Stress (The PILOTS Database) <www.ncptsd.org>*** **2000**
- ***Referativnyi Zhurnal (Abstracts Journal of the All-Russian Institute of Scientific and Technical Information–in Russian)*** **2000**

Special Bibliographic Notes related to special journal issues (separates) and indexing/abstracting:

- indexing/abstracting services in this list will also cover material in any "separate" that is co-published simultaneously with Haworth's special thematic journal issue or DocuSerial. Indexing/abstracting usually covers material at the article/chapter level.
- monographic co-editions are intended for either non-subscribers or libraries which intend to purchase a second copy for their circulating collections.
- monographic co-editions are reported to all jobbers/wholesalers/approval plans. The source journal is listed as the "series" to assist the prevention of duplicate purchasing in the same manner utilized for books-in-series.
- to facilitate user/access services all indexing/abstracting services are encouraged to utilize the co-indexing entry note indicated at the bottom of the first page of each article/chapter/contribution.
- this is intended to assist a library user of any reference tool (whether print, electronic, online, or CD-ROM) to locate the monographic version if the library has purchased this version but not a subscription to the source journal.

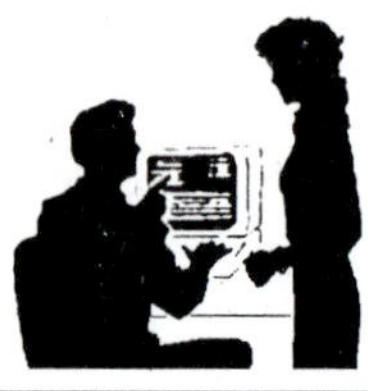

Trauma and Sexuality: The Effects of Childhood Sexual, Physical, and Emotional Abuse on Sexual Identity and Behavior

CONTENTS

COMMENTARY

ABOUT THE EDITORS

James A. Chu, MD, is Chief of Hospital Clinical Services at McLean Hospital in Belmont, Massachusetts, and Associate Professor of Psychiatry at Harvard Medical School. He is widely known for his clinical work, teaching, and research concerning the post-traumatic effects of childhood trauma. As a teacher, Dr. Chu is known for his empathic and pragmatic approach to understanding and treating survivors of childhood abuse. His publications in the psychiatric literature include both basic research on the effects of childhood abuse and discussions concerning the nature and techniques of treatment of abuse survivors. Dr. Chu is a Fellow of the American Psychiatric Association and the International Society for the Study of Dissociation. In addition, he is the recipient of the ISSD's Cornelia B. Wilbur Award and Distinguished Achievement Awards for outstanding contributions in the field of dissociative disorders and the Pierre Janet Writing Award for his 1998 book *Rebuilding Shattered Lives*, published by John Wiley & Sons.

Elizabeth S. Bowman, MD, is Clinical Professor of Neurology and former Professor of Psychiatry at the Indiana University School of Medicine. In addition, she is Attending Psychiatrist at Indiana University Hospitals and Consulting Psychiatrist for the University Hospital's Epilepsy Clinic. She is the author or co-author of numerous journal articles and book chapters, and has presented papers at national and international conferences. Dr. Bowman is the recipient of three Teaching Awards from Indiana University, as well as the winner of the President's Award of Distinction from the International Society for the Study of Dissociation. She is also listed in all four editions of the *Best Doctors in America*. Dr. Bowman is former president of the Indiana Psychiatric Society, a member of the American Medical Women's Association, Association of Women Psychiatrists, member and Fellow of the American Psychiatric Association and Fellow and former president of the International Society for the Study of Dissociation.

∞ ALL HAWORTH MEDICAL PRESS BOOKS
AND JOURNALS ARE PRINTED
ON CERTIFIED ACID-FREE PAPER

Introduction: Trauma and Sexuality: The Effects of Childhood Sexual, Physical, and Emotional Abuse on Adult Sexual Identity and Behavior

In the modern era of trauma studies, we, as clinicians and researchers, have been treating and investigating the effects of trauma–including the sexual abuse of children–for more than 20 years. And yet, we know far more about sequelae such as post-traumatic and dissociative symptoms, disrupted attachment, addictions, eating disorders, and somatoform symptoms than we do about the effects of trauma on sexual behavior. With the exception of relatively few articles in the scientific literature (many of which were written by the authors in this collection of papers), little has been hypothesized or studied about the sexual effects of sexual abuse and other childhood maltreatment.

Why have we neglected this obvious and important area? Perhaps the reason can be simply attributed to our Victorian legacy of reluctance to openly discuss sexuality despite the reality of all humans being innately sexual beings and having sexual lives and fantasies. Or, perhaps the reason may be related to some of the expressions of sexuality that are sometimes seen in persons with childhood trauma. Expressions such as sexual addiction, homosexuality, sadomasochistic behavior, and prostitution have been at times classified as deviant and this may have contributed to our reluctance to discuss them openly. Or, perhaps the reason

[Haworth co-indexing entry note]: "Introduction: Trauma and Sexuality: The Effects of Childhood Sexual, Physical, and Emotional Abuse on Adult Sexual Identity and Behavior." Chu, James A., and Elizabeth S. Bowman. Co-published simultaneously in *Journal of Trauma & Dissociation* (The Haworth Medical Press, an imprint of The Haworth Press, Inc.) Vol. 3, No. 4, 2002, pp. 1-4; and: *Trauma and Sexuality: The Effects of Childhood Sexual, Physical, and Emotional Abuse on Sexuality Identity and Behavior* (ed: James A. Chu, and Elizabeth S. Bowman) The Haworth Medical Press, an imprint of The Haworth Press, Inc., 2002, pp. 1-4. Single or multiple copies of this article are available for a fee from The Haworth Document Delivery Service [1-800-HAWORTH, 9:00 a.m. - 5:00 p.m. (EST). E-mail address: getinfo@haworthpressinc.com].

is that we collectively wish to deny the effects of abuse on one of the core aspects of ourselves–to deny that early traumatic events forever change the sexual lives of persons in such an intimate and profound way.

Elizabeth Howell in " 'Good Girls,' Sexy 'Bad Girls,' and Warriors: The Role of Trauma and Dissociation in the Creation and Reproduction of Gender," proposes a theory concerning gender–that "femininity" and "masculinity," the personality styles in our culture, are direct and indirect outcomes of trauma and reflective of dissociation. Her article delineates various ways that trauma may be an important contributing factor to the formation of gendered states and sexual behaviors both in healthy and pathological adaptations. Dr. Howell notes differing patterns for females and males that reflect social norms, stereotypical child-rearing patterns, and biological predispositions that are shaped by the effects of trauma.

Margo Rivera has been a pioneer in the area of trauma treatment with persons who have non-heterosexual sexual orientation. Her paper, "Informed and Supportive Treatment for Lesbian, Gay, Bisexual and Transgendered Trauma Survivors," is a comprehensive review of the need to address sexuality as part of treatment, and a reminder that there is a wide range of healthy expressions of sexuality and gender. Dr. Rivera points out that clients who are not heterosexual require a therapeutic context in which their expression of gender identity and sexual orientation are acknowledged and clearly supported. The psychotherapeutic process must emphasize the ability to live freely and fully, and must counteract their sense of being disenfranchised both as abused children and as adults with an alternative sexual orientation.

The paper by Steven Gold and Robert Seifer, "Dissociation and Sexual Addiction/Compulsivity: A Contextual Approach to Conceptualization and Treatment," explores the relationship of dissociation to sexual addiction/compulsivity in childhood sexual abuse survivors. Their clinical observations have led them to argue that it is essential to recognize the dissociative quality of sexual addiction/compulsivity in childhood sexual abuse survivors in order to treat the sexual dysfunction. The authors also propose that sexual addiction/compulsivity may reflect the dissociated reenactments of early relational disturbances, resulting in difficulties with integration of sexual activity with appropriate affective states. A treatment model is discussed that includes attention to not only dysfunctional sexual behavior, but also to dissociation and relational contextual issues.

Toni Cavanagh Johnson addresses a sensitive and critical issue in her paper, "Some Considerations About Sexual Abuse and Children with Sexual Behavior Problems." She discusses and delineates three groups of children who engage in problematic sexual behavior, only one of which is molesting other children, She notes the diversity of reasons for the development of problematic sexual behavior, and refutes the belief that sexually abused children are destined to go on to molest others. Dr. Johnson points out the importance of distinguishing between children who engage in natural and healthy sexual behaviors, sexually-reactive behaviors, extensive but mutual sexual behaviors, and children who molest. Her paper and the outcome statistics that she summarizes are an important antidote to the popular and destructive myth that the abused are inevitably destined to become abusers. Dr. Johnson's categories of sexual behaviors in children are a useful guide for clinicians who evaluate child survivors of sexual abuse.

Mark Schwartz and Lori Galperin's paper, "Hyposexuality and Hypersexuality Secondary to Childhood Trauma and Dissociation," discusses the effect of childhood trauma on the capacity of survivors for adult sexual activity and intimacy. They draw on the disruption of essential childhood relational attachments and early dissociative reactions that have systematic effects on arousal, desire and pair-bonding. The authors describe a treatment model that addresses the early trauma and its aftereffects concerning intimacy and sexuality.

The study by Cheryl Gore-Felton and Cheryl Koopman, "Traumatic Experiences: Harbinger of Risk Behavior Among HIV-Positive Adults," examines the relationship between trauma history, trauma-related symptoms, and sexual risk behavior. Investigating whether early abuse was related to later sexual risk behavior, these authors found that moderate to severe trauma symptoms were significantly correlated with unprotected sexual intercourse. Intrusive trauma symptoms correlated significantly with having multiple partners, and intrusive and avoidant symptoms were associated with unprotected sex. Overall, greater intrusive symptoms and less avoidant symptoms were positively associated with greater sexual risk behavior. The authors hypothesize that reducing trauma symptoms among affected adults might be a particularly effective HIV-prevention intervention.

In his commentary, "Sexual Orientation Conflict in the Dissociative Disorders," Colin Ross raises the issue of a greater than expected proportion of gay and lesbian patients in his trauma program. This phenomenon has been observed in other similar programs, but no one has systematically explored it, perhaps due to the complex and contradictory questions it raises, e.g., does sexual abuse of girls by male perpetrators result in aversion to heterosexual intimacy, while sexual abuse of boys by male perpetrators predispose them to a homosexual identification? Dr. Ross has formulated the questions about this and other politically sensitive topics and challenges all of us to begin to find answers.

These authors have done much to rectify the relative absence of discussion and knowledge in the area of trauma and sexuality. Their contributions are expressions of intellectual curiosity, solid scientific inquiry, and the courage to address sensitive areas. In doing so, they help us expand our sensitivity and expertise in a critically important way. They help us look non-judgmentally at the profound effects of long-standing early abuse on the sexual identities, orientation, behaviors, and fantasies of those who we seek to help. If we cannot help the traumatized patients that we treat in all domains of their lives–including their sexuality–we have failed in our attempts to help them to become truly restored in adapting to healthy lives.

James A. Chu, MD
Elizabeth S. Bowman, MD

"Good Girls," Sexy "Bad Girls," and Warriors: The Role of Trauma and Dissociation in the Creation and Reproduction of Gender

Elizabeth F. Howell, PhD

SUMMARY. The thesis of this article is that substantially, "femininity" and "masculinity," the gendered personality styles so common in our culture, are direct and indirect outcomes of trauma, and reflective of dissociation. In addition to being direct sequellae of trauma, these "post-traumatic styles" may become consensually accepted modes of interaction by virtue of vicarious and anticipatory trauma. The patterns tend to differ for females and males, reflecting social forces, including sex-typed child-rearing patterns, and biological predispositions interacting with trauma. While presenting self-states of abused girls and women often tend to be compliant, childlike, passive, masochistic, "good," vulnerable, sweet, and dependent–characteristics often considered stereotypical for females, posttraumatic aggressivity of boys may appear indistinguishable from stereotypical "masculinity." Aggressivity and

Elizabeth F. Howell is affiliated with the Department of Psychology, New York University, New York, NY.

Address correspondence to: Elizabeth F. Howell, PhD, 111 Hicks Street, #5P, Brooklyn, NY 11201 (E-mail: efhowell@aol.com).

The author wishes to thank Carol Kemelgor, ACSW, Ruth Blizard, PhD, Shielagh Shusta, PhD, as well as the anonymous reviewers for their careful reading and helpful comments.

[Haworth co-indexing entry note]: " 'Good Girls,' Sexy 'Bad Girls,' and Warriors: The Role of Trauma and Dissociation in the Creation and Reproduction of Gender." Howell, Elizabeth F. Co-published simultaneously in *Journal of Trauma & Dissociation* (The Haworth Medical Press, an imprint of The Haworth Press, Inc.) Vol. 3, No. 4, 2002, pp. 5-32; and: *Trauma and Sexuality: The Effects of Childhood Sexual, Physical, and Emotional Abuse on Sexuality Identity and Behavior* (ed: James A. Chu, and Elizabeth S. Bowman) The Haworth Medical Press, an imprint of The Haworth Press, Inc., 2002, pp. 5-32. Single or multiple copies of this article are available for a fee from The Haworth Document Delivery Service [1-800-HAWORTH, 9:00 a.m. - 5:00 p.m. (EST). E-mail address: getinfo@haworthpressinc.com].

violence reproduce trauma, which then contributes to the reproduction of gender.

KEYWORDS. Abuse, dissociation, femininity, gender, masculinity, stereotypes, trauma

This article will propose a trauma- and dissociation-based theory for the creation and reproduction of gender. The thesis will be developed that, substantially, "femininity" and "masculinity," the gendered personality styles so common in our culture, are direct and indirect outcomes of trauma and reflective of dissociation. Most of the literature on gender omits the effects of trauma and dissociation. The article delineates some different ways that trauma may be an important contributing factor to the formation of gendered states and behaviors, especially pathological ones, in males and females. However, the presence of gendered characteristics in a given individual should in no way be taken as *prima facie* evidence that trauma or abuse has occurred.

TRAUMA HAS BEEN LEFT OUT OF ACADEMIC GENDER STUDIES

In our culture, sex and gender categorizations are probably the most basic in organizing human life (Bem, 1983). Accounting for gender has been important to feminist men and women because gender and beliefs about gender, in addition to being all-pervasive, have markedly limited women's access to social and economic power, and because prescriptive gender has also limited the full self-expression of human beings. The assumed superiority of males not only endangers, harms, and devalues women, but it devalues all that is female-associated, thus engendering fears in men about not measuring up to standards of masculinity.

Various subdisciplines in the social sciences and mental health have offered a multitude of theories of the origins of gender. Especially notable among these are psychoanalytic theory, social learning theory, cognitive developmental theory, gender schema theory, biological theories, social constructionism, theories of public versus private spheres,

Chodorow's (1974, 1978) theory of gender differentiation on the basis of differing mother-daughter and mother-son dynamics, Gilligan's theory (Gilligan, 1982; Gilligan & Attanuccu, 1988) of the "different voice" which is partially based on Chodorow's theory, Belenky, Clinchy, Goldberger and Tarule's (1986) theory of "women's ways of knowing," the "self-in-relation" theory of Jordan, Kaplan, Miller, Stiver, and Surry (1991) of the Stone Center at Wellesley College, and Maccoby's (1990) theory of children's peer group interactions. Some of these theories are contradictory to each other in their assertions and points of view about human development. Remarkably few of the theories of gender assess trauma. And, trauma may be the touchstone for understanding the gender configurations.

While our theories of gender have recognized the pathology of gender prescriptions, they have failed to discriminate aspects of gendered behavior that are clearly pathological from those that are not necessarily so, e.g., passivity and masochism in females and narcissism and hyper-aggressivity in males. The thesis of this paper is that much of "gendered" behavior and experience, especially the pathological aspects, is, in interaction with other forces, trauma-generated; and that it is the post-traumatic and dissociated aspects of this gendered behavior that makes it so resistant to change. When one views gender stereotypes (such as men are independent, active, tough, unemotional, and violent, and women are dependent, passive, emotional, and caring) through the prism of trauma, the bifurcation of typology along dominant/submissive lines becomes immediately evident. As a case in point, consider Freud's male, masculine, active, aggressive, dominant, and female, feminine, passive, submissive, masochistic categorizations (Schafer, 1974). Trauma and dissociation tend to shatter subjectivity and agency, forcing the person into dominant/submissive modalities of thinking and behavior.

The rates of child trauma in this country continue to be unacceptably high (Chu, 1998, 2001). The hypothesis presented in this paper is that different patterns of child trauma experienced by boys and girls, along with their broader repercussions, correspond to the different patterns of gendered behavior and experience. Indeed, some of the stereotypic norms may reflect posttraumatic states and affects that have been normalized. On the whole, boys are more often victims of physical violence (Boney-McCoy & Finkelhor, 1995), while girls are more often subject to sexual abuse (Finkelhor & Dsiuba-Leatherman, 1994). The patterns of child sexual abuse also differ for boys and girls, such that boys, more than girls, tend to be abused outside of the home by extrafamilial persons (Finkelhor, 1990). The gender of the perpetrators also varies: while males are the most frequent perpetrators for both boys and girls, the male/female ratio is higher for girls. In a large study involving interviews of 900 women, Russell (1986) found a prevalence of contact child sexual abuse of girls before the age of 18 of 38%, and of incest, a rate of 16%. Ninety percent (90%) of the abusers were male. Results of Lisak, Hopper, and Song's (1996) study of 600 college men indicated that while 34% of the men reported physical abuse as children, 18% reported contact sexual abuse before the age of sixteen, with 3-4% of that being incestuous. Sixty-one percent (61%) of the sexual abusers were male and 28% were female, while 11% of the boys had both male and female abusers. Cumulative date indicate that girls are at least two times (Finkelhor, 1990), in some studies, three times (Little & Hamby, 1999) as likely to be subjected to sexual abuse as are boys. An extrapolation from the above figures would indicate that girls are about four times as likely to be subjected to incest. However, it should be borne in mind that self-report measures, especially self-report measures of boys' sexual abuse, may be underestimates (Gartner, 1999; Little & Hamby, 1999). Furthermore, definitions of incest and child sexual abuse may vary with investigator. Child sexual abuse is a broad category including vast differences in type, chronicity, and severity (Benatar, 2000).

While both sexes are subject to violence and harm, some of the ways in which boys and girls are harmed vary by gender. Crime statistics indicate that boys are subject to much more homicide and assault while girls are greatly more subject to rape (Finkelhor, 1990). A recent national survey, conducted by telephone, of 2000 randomly selected youths, aged 10-16 (Boney-McCoy & Finkelhor, 1995) found that about one half (47.4%) of the boys had been subjected to some form of violent victimization, as compared to one third of the girls. About twice as many girls had been subject to attempted kidnapping. Taken together over 40% of these children had been victimized. (Only 5.7% of these incidents had been reported to the police, and about one quarter had never been disclosed to anyone before the survey.) Again, patterns were found to vary in and out of the home: a slightly higher percentage of girls than boys had been subject to parental and family assault than boys; but the boys had been exposed to about three times as much aggravated assault and simple assault by non-family members than the girls. A follow-up, prospective, longitudinal study, which controlled for the quality of the parent-child relationship, found that both male and female participants who had been victimized, experienced more PTSD symptoms than those who had not. In addition, perhaps in consonance with the idea that boys, even little ones, should be "tough," boys, much more than girls, tend to be subject to a potentially traumatic premature separation from their mothers (Pollack, 1998).

In order to support and clarify my thesis, I will first cover some background, including the differentiation of "gender" from "sex," and the prevailing theories and politics in academic feminist psychology. Following this, I will delineate what I see as the posttraumatic gendering of girls and boys: (1) the girls' picture, (2) the boys' picture, (3) Bruce Perry's contribution, and (4) the reproduction of gender.

BACKGROUND: GENDER AND THE DIVIDED FEMINIST AGENDA

Originally a word denoting "kind" (genus, genre, generic) and used in some languages to classify nouns and pronouns by sex (Pinker, 1994), the term, "gender," has been adopted by feminists to make a needed conceptual distinction between the effects of biology and culture. Having had only one word, "sex" made it difficult to understand and talk about behavior that is sex-typed but culturally mediated. It also led to circular thinking: even though we may know that behavior is influenced by situations, context, and history, without a word to designate this knowledge, it is easy to confuse sex and gender, and especially to ascribe the effects of the latter to the former, thereby reducing gendered behaviors to a biological essence dictated by genes and hormones.

Until very, very recently, women have usually been represented in the mental health field and other disciplines as deficient in one important way or another, and therefore deserving of reduced status relative to men (Hare-Mustin & Marecek, 1990; Kemelgor & Etzowitz, 2000; Unger, 1990). In the social sciences, there has been a divided feminist response to the *homme manqué* model of the female, one minimizing gender differences in order to de-emphasize the alleged deficiency, and one which maximized, but valorized them (Bohan, 1993; Hare-Mustin & Marecek, 1990). Many feminist social scientists in the first group have concentrated their efforts on showing that men and women are not markedly different, and that what we see as gender is largely a cultural and social artifact. This agenda has had mixed success, depending upon what particular kinds of differences are being considered, and by whom. A second group of feminist psychologists, often known as the "cultural feminists" including writers such as Jean Baker Miller and

Carol Gilligan (Bohan, 1993; Mednick, 1989; Hare-Mustin & Marecek, 1990), have revalued the earlier devalued "feminine" characteristics. Jean Baker Miller, author of the groundbreaking *Toward a New Psychology of Women* (1976), recategorized women's service and relational orientation, as strength rather than as weakness; and later, she and her colleagues (1991) at the Stone Center at Wellesley College promulgated the "self-in-relation" theory of female psychology. Six years after the publication of Miller's book, Carol Gilligan's highly acclaimed *In a Different Voice* (1982) appeared, presenting one of the more popular, if not the most popular current theory about the origins of gender differences. She claimed that women and girls' often overlooked relationality is, in fact, an often unheard or misunderstood "different voice." Grounding her presentation of the genders in Nancy Chodorow's (1974, 1978) work and in Lawrence Kohlberg's (1966) cognitive developmental theory, Gilligan proposed that girls and women follow a "care" orientation, a path of cognitive/moral development, that differs from the "justice" oriented moral developmental path that she considered more characteristic of males. Two important criticisms of this strand of feminist thinking have been (1) that it may give support to the stereotypes of femininity, legitimizing the patriarchal status quo, and (2) that it is an essentialist point of view, conceptualizing gender as an inherent, immutable, and indelible aspect of self (Bohan, 1993; Mednick, 1989). Nonetheless, the theory resonates with the experience of many people, especially women, of themselves and others.

Perhaps one reason for this resonance is that peoples' experience is embedded in context. An impressive array of social psychological studies has illustrated the ways in which gender is determined by context. Women and men, as roughly separate groups, tend to find themselves in differing situations that differentially elicit "feminine" and "masculine" behaviors. This can lead to the perception that gender refers to enduring and stable traits that are either learned or are linked to a biological substrate that determines feminine and masculine behavior. Much social psychological research indicates that a great deal of the "gender" ascribed to people may be more "in" the situations that they inhabit, than "in" them (Unger, 1990). From this point of view, Gilligan's (1982) thesis about the female caring orientation may be understood as a reflection of context–that women are more frequently in situations that elicit or demand caring. When men are in similar situations, they may be just as caring (Clopton & Sorrell, 1993; Mednick, 1989). Furthermore, more recent moral development research has indicated that males do not score higher than females on Kohlberg's moral development scale

(Braebeck, 1989; Gilligan & Attanucci, 1988). From my point of view, the most important contribution of Gilligan's and others' uncovering of the caring orientation is in the importance of nurturing a caring orientation in both sexes.

Oppression is a powerful context as well as an ongoing source of socialization. There has been a voluminous literature on the relationship between gender and oppression, an exegesis of which is beyond the scope of this paper. The correspondence between so-called "feminine" behaviors and that of subordinate, oppressed groups has been variously and compellingly described by Allport (1954), Brown (1992), de Beauvoir (1953), Dinnerstein (1976), Espin and Gawalek (1992), Friedan (1963), Giddings (1984), Hacker (1981), Hooks (1984, 1989), Horney (1934), Hurtado (1989), Landrine (1989), Lerman (1986), Lerner (1982), Mill (1972/1869), Shainess (1970) and Thompson (1964), among many others. Because gender is so endemically interwoven with daily life, gender-linked oppression is inescapable. In particular, psychological self-oppression resulting from the internalization of sexist mores and stereotypes, such as that described by Hacker, Horney, and Thompson, is an important aspect of the reproduction of gender.

While oppressive circumstances contribute to the socialization and perpetuation of gendered behavior, they also tend to be traumatogenic. As Brown (1991), Herman (1992), and Root (1992) observe, the frequency with which females are exposed to trauma (and the kinds of trauma) are not "outside the range" of the normative, and the impact of trauma upon psychic life and psychopathology is considerable. Accordingly, it may often be the trauma, rather than the oppression, per se, that substantially mediates many gendered conditions. Oppression, especially behavioral oppression, that is, the exercise of overt power, is not of necessity traumatic–that is, overwhelming and exceeding the mind's capacity to register it, rendering the person helpless to understand. My thesis is that much of the behavior we think of as gendered is derivative of trauma specifically, that specifically "gendered" (typed) self states are created by trauma. These include "the good girl," the sexy "bad girl" in females and "warrior" states in males, among others. Gendering is a multipart and multi-layered process. Because child trauma is so ubiquitous and frequent, these behaviors become labeled and codified. Because the types of traumatic experience tend to be distributed in accordance with biological sex, these labels tend to cohere with the (usually patriarchal) social structure, and become gender stereotypes.

Regardless of whether or how much stereotypes represent bias in the observer, or actual behavior in the observed, they tend to be internalized in psychic life, where they can become gender role standards (Howell, 1975) serving as modulators of self-esteem (shame and guilt), thereby influencing behavior. The gender-socialized individual is now situated as a player in a social process that depends upon gender-related prior learning and training, involves gender-related contextual demands, unconscious self-monitoring, and the high possibility of past and future trauma.

Trauma is by definition overwhelming, changing physiology, cognition, and emotion. The core of trauma is the experience of being rendered completely helpless (Spiegel, 1990). Without the opportunity to heal wounds, mourn, and reconfigure interpersonal dynamics, trauma tends to be reenacted. Reflecting patterns of adaptation to and identification with the aggressor, complementary submissive and dominant, masochistic and sadistic states may exist, alternating within and between individuals (Blizard, 2001; Howell, in press). These states are not inherently masculine or feminine; but they tend, as a result of the combination and interaction of various forces, including socialization, trauma, and sex-differentiated biological predispositions, to be disproportionately distributed among males and females. Elsewhere (Howell, in press) I have described my view of how trauma creates abuser/sadistic states and victim/masochistic states. The former derives from experience of being so dependent upon the abuser and the abuser's state of mind that one is "taken over" by an identification with the abuser (Coates & Moore, 1995), and the latter is based in part upon the person's own "freeze" state (Nijenhuis, Vanderlinden, & Spinhoven, 1998) as victim. Both states exist in traumatized people, but they tend to shift within and between people. Part of this alternation is dependent upon projection into others and into parts of the self. These psychodynamics, in conjunction with traumatic circumstance, social structure, socialization patterns and genetic predispositions, contribute to generally different types of enactments in accordance with sex. This may microcosmically represent in individual survivors the power dynamics of the larger culture, in particular, the ways that gender tends to coincide with a power/powerless, dominance/submission binary (Rivera, 1989).

While these states are in themselves neither male nor female, sometimes highly dissociated self-states are distinctly gender-linked. In particular, the process of identification with the abuser may replicate the abuser's gender identity/and or sexual orientation, injecting confusion in some survivors about their own gender identity and sexual orientation (Layton, 1998). Thus, in our clinical populations we may find, for example, a self-identified heterosexual man, who was repeatedly abused by an uncle, and who at times compulsively seeks homosexual liaisons; a self-identified heterosexual man who was abused by his mother, and who has a seductive female part; females who were abused by males and who have male parts; females who were abused by females and who have lesbian parts (Blizard, 1997). None of the foregoing is meant to imply that childhood abuse causes homosexuality. In cases where abusers were of both sexes, there may be an overriding general confusion about gender identity and sexual orientation, such that we can only extrapolate that the gender of some of the self-states is probably based upon the gender of the perpetrator.

The above is a view that, to a significant extent, the highly gendered psyche, especially in its pathological aspects, may be a fragmented, unintegrated one. Gender roles and gendered states end up "containing" trauma, keeping knowledge of and outrage about trauma out of awareness and perpetuating it all at the same time. As reenactment, gender repeats itself interpersonally, socially, and transgenerationally.

Most of the foregoing speaks to the social construction of gender. Recently, Copjec (1994) has introduced a formulation of the later Lacanian concept of the Real in terms of gender. This has to do with the way in which trauma is itself unknowable and unrepresentable. She depicts a view of gender in terms of "the impossibility of meaning" (Dyess & Dean, 2000; Stern, 2000) rather than the possibility of many meanings posed by social constructivism. Trauma punctures the psyche; the hole or "lack" is itself unknowable, unsymbolizable. We can only infer it in terms of its aftereffects. In accordance with the view that trauma contributes substantially to gender, and that the two are intensely interrelated, the gendered psyche may not only be a fragmented one, but a punctured one; and this combination may contribute to the particular recalcitrance of gender to change.

Finally, a last objection to the caring orientation: caring and tenderness need to be distinguished from passivity, dependency, and masochism. The caring orientation in itself fails to explain the latter characteristics, which are not necessarily "caring" at all. The alternative presented here is that certain part of stereotypical femininity, the pathological part, is substantially trauma generated. Likewise, hyperaggressivity and pathological narcissism in men, need to be distinguished from healthy self-esteem and from healthy aggression that protects self and others.

THE POSTTRAUMATIC GENDERING OF GIRLS AND BOYS

The Girls' Picture

It is my hypothesis that a portion of the gender stereotypic cultural norms for females derives directly and indirectly from the susceptibility of girls to be sexually abused and/or narcissistically used as sex objects, directly from the impact of trauma, and indirectly from other sources, as will be described. This certainly fits with the pattern that Brown and Gilligan (1992) as well as Belenky and her colleagues (1986) observe that girls tend to lose their voices in early adolescence. Sexually abused girls are often instructed to lose their voices, that is: "Don't tell."

Implicit in the caring orientation is emphasis upon the importance of attachments. While awareness of attachment may directly underlie some of the commonly gendered characteristics such as *emotionality* and *nurturance*, attachment in itself is not sufficient to generate a fuller list of gendered characteristics that would include *masochistic*, *dependent*, *passive*, etc. It is in the interaction between attachment and trauma/dissociation, in particular, in the configurations that emerge when attachment, especially to an abusive caretaker, becomes markedly more important than the person's own agendas and desires, that female gendering begins to take a fuller conventional form.

Among the sequellae of child sex abuse are mental states that exemplify some of the common stereotypes: the feminine linked passivity, dependency, masochism, helplessness, and seductive or highly sexual states as well as the masculine linked tough-guy, violent, and rageful (Rivera, 1989; Shusta, 1999). Trauma can fracture the person into various self-states along the lines of dominant-subordinate, predator-prey relationships. The feminine gendered form of these may fall into divisions of the "good girl" and the sexualized "bad girl," corresponding to an age-old Madonna/whore split. The "good girl" is socially acceptable, and is perhaps the template for some of the usual academic lists of stereotypes, such as passivity, dependency, emotionality, excitability, talkativeness, indecisiveness, insecurity, suggestibility, illogicalness, intuitiveness, affectionateness, tempermentalness (Broverman, Broverman, Clarkson, Rosenkrantz, & Vogel, 1972).

The "Good Girl"

In psychopathology, whether the clinical outcome is dissociative identity disorder (DID), borderline personality disorder (BPD), or what we think of as neurosis characterized by intrapsychic conflict and compromise formation, the usual presenting self-state (usually a version of "the good girl") tends to be drained and depleted of life, relatively helpless, depressed, masochistic and feminine-identified, in females. Certainly, females with DID may have male gendered parts, and females with BPD can have self-states that are explosively angry and violent. However, the posttraumatic states that are most frequently visible to others and available to usual conscious experience are predictably those that were most adjusted to the power dynamics of the social context of early life, and possibly the present one as well.

The other-orientation, so often described as characteristic of females, may amount to a "gendered subjectivity" according to which females are required to always respond to someone else's needs (Miller, 1976; Profitt, 2001). As Gilligan (1982) states about the conventional stage, a stage in which girls and women are most often caught:

> Here the conventional feminine voice emerges with great clarity, defining the self and proclaiming its worth on the basis of the ability to care for and protect others. The woman now constructs a world perfused with the assumptions about feminine goodness that are reflected in the stereotypes of the Broverman et al. studies (1972), where all the attributes considered desirable for women presume an other–the recipient of (such qualities as tact, gentleness, and emotional expressiveness) which allow the woman to respond sensitively while evoking in return the care (of the recipient). . . . (p. 79)

The other-orientedness described here may be less extreme, but not so different in kind, from that of the abused female child, who feels herself into the mind and body of her abuser in order to stay alive (Ferenczi, 1949). Her mental and emotional activity is focused on the welfare of her abuser, because her welfare depends on his state of mind, and on his being pleased with her.

The Sexy "Bad Girl"

Compulsive seductive sexuality and/or the inability to refuse sexual advances (cf., Freyd's "consensual sex decision mechanism" (1996)), including prostitution, are not infrequent outcomes of child sexual abuse (Davies & Frawley, 1994; Schetky, 1990). This is not the kind of sexuality that is characterized by vitality and high self-esteem. As

Ferenczi (1949) observed about the consequences of child sexual abuse in "Confusion of Tongues":

> When subjected to sexual attack, under the pressure of such traumatic urgency, the child can develop instantaneously all the emotions of mature adults and all the potential qualities dormant in him that normally belong to marriage, maternity and fatherhood. One is justified–in contradistinction to the familiar regression–to speak of a *traumatic progression*, of a *precocious maturity*. It is natural to compare this with the precocious maturity of the fruit that was injured by a bird or insect. . . . the sexually abused child may become "a guilty love-automaton imitating the adult anxiously, self-effacingly. (pp. 229-230)

Coinciding with the split between the "good girl" and the sexy "bad girl" that can exist in some individual psyches, is one in the popular imagination. Another aspect of the "bad girl, fallen woman" aspect of femininity is the *femme fatale*. Consider the interpersonal dynamics involved: the *femme fatale* enslaves men, reversing her own earlier traumatic enslavement, e.g., Odysseus's Circe, the "black widow," "the vamp," movies such as *Cat People*, *Black Widow*, *The Last Seduction*, and so on. The *femme fatale* is always reenacting trauma. Indeed, reenactment of trauma is both her *modus operandi* and her *raison d'etre*. Such compulsivity is characteristic of a posttraumatic state which reenacts abuse. The *femme fatale* understands this reenacting state to be female.

Rage

It is dangerous for subordinated and terrorized people to show rage, especially at the time of trauma. Lott (1990) has observed that, in contrast to an angry voice, the caring voice, considered characteristic of females, may be the only voice the male world will recognize. Rage, which tends to be male-associated, is generally considered unattractive, "unfeminine" in women. For many women rage is suppressed, repressed–or dissociated. Although this may vary with subculture, women with Borderline Personality Disorder (BPD) may frequently exhibit violent, explosive rage states all the while disavowing these states and maintaining a view of themselves as always meek and mild. In females with Dissociative Identity Disorders the aggressor, protector states are frequently male gendered. As Rivera (1988) observes, "Through creating personalities who declared themselves male, they were able to identify with the aggression of their abusers and use it in the service of their own protection without consciously challenging their socialization as girls and women" (p. 44).

Vicarious Trauma and Indirect Effects of Trauma

Perhaps a good portion of the girls who have not themselves been abused have witnessed abuse to another person, such as a sibling, parent, relative, or friend. They may simply know that as girls they are vulnerable (Waites, 1993). Such vicarious trauma will probably not cause the fragmentation that may be generated within the victims, but it can create fear. Just as the trauma of the Holocaust can be transmitted intergenerationally (Danieli, 1985), the trauma of child sex abuse may possibly be similarly passed on, as well. As a case example, a mother who was herself incested as a child, attempted to protect her daughter by instructing her to "watch out" for the dangers of abuse that she, herself, had been unable to avoid. Possibly the warning did help her daughter, but possibly some of the mother's paralysis was transmitted as well, for the daughter reports that when it did happen that she was sexually violated as an adult by an acquaintance, she felt helpless to resist and laughed nervously in response to the abuser's behavior. Remarkably, when told of the occurrence by her daughter, the mother uttered a similar nervous laugh. While only the mother had been subjected to the childhood trauma, the daughter also was perhaps subject to a replication of the posttraumatic response, despite the warning. The "warning" may have carried with it the additional messages of the futility of struggle, confrontation, and self-defense.

Thus, while direct sexual abuse is not the lot of the majority of girls, its threat is pervasive. Girls often know about it from their family members and friends. Even without direct physical contact, verbally incestuous remarks can be damaging to self-esteem and a person's sense of safety and security. While a few such remarks may not, in themselves, be overwhelming, in sufficient quantity, with a certain intonation, and as part of a general atmosphere–particularly in combination with other trauma and/or neglect, they may amount to a cumulative trauma. Root (1992) classifies these indirect effects of trauma as "insidious trauma."

The above is not intended to be a sweeping claim along the lines of Brownmiller's (1975) assertion that rape is a process of intimidation by "which *all* men keep *all* women in a state of fear" (p. 15). I agree with Asher (1988) that, "The effect of sexual abuse serves to increase the power of men over women and to create women who simultaneously fear men, overvalue and overidealize men because of their immense power, and are dependent on them" (p. 15). Along with sexual harassment which directly affects approximately 50% of girls and women (Fitzgerald, 1993), rape that has at least a 14% prevalence (Koss, 1993) and battering, child sexual abuse both reflects and reinforces girls' and women's' lower status. In contrast to the above-mentioned experiences, some of which are shattering even to adults (cf., Raine, 1998), child sexual abuse can affect the developing child much more powerfully. Taken together these potentialities may constitute an unformulated nucleus of concern, around which contagious anxiety and social consciousness organize. Emotional resonances to this nucleus may be evoked by intergenerationally transmitted anxiety around trauma and concurrent vicarious traumatization.

How would these characteristics of passivity, dependency, masochism, and helplessness that may reflect trauma become gender stereotypical? The "caring orientation" is two-sided. Jean Baker Miller (1976) states that what women want is to serve without being subservient. Mature caring and attachment need are often conflated, and their respective implications need to be differentiated. Certainly autonomous, self-selected service is the most desirable way to serve, but the other side of the caring orientation–the side without autonomy, is masochism and passivity. The "dark side" of the caring orientation is the other-orientation of terrified subjugation and devaluation.

The Boys' Picture

The typography most often cited for prescriptive stereotypical masculinity is Brannon's (1976) description of four clusters of norms for masculinity: the Sturdy Oak (which emphasizes physical strength and emotional fortitude), Big Wheel (emphasizing success and achievement), Give 'em Hell (aggression), and No Sissy Stuff (masculinity is avoidance of anything feminine). Various writers in men's studies have their own focus on the problematic "gender straight-jacket" in which boys are raised (Pollack, 1998), but it is generally acknowledged that deviance from gender role prescriptions and proscriptions has more severe consequences for males than for females. (Pleck, 1995; Unger and Crawford, 1995). Men are often described as being unemotional in outward behavior. Indeed, Levant claims that there is "a high incidence among men of at least a mild form of alexithymia–the inability to identify and describe one's feelings in words" (1995, p. 238). Despite this, measures of physiological responsivity indicate emotionality equal to that of women (Pollack, 1998). Men are often less practiced in expressing their feelings, which may then be channeled into anger (Pollack, 1998; Kilmartin, 1991; Levant, 1995). Many authors in men's studies emphasize the general unacceptability of expression of emotions, other than anger. Especially forbidden are feelings of loss, vulnerability, and shame. In contrast to females, who are more often shame sensitive, boys tend to be "shame phobic" (Pollack, 1998, p. 33). As a result, narcissistic defenses may be overdeveloped. (Betcher & Pollack, 1993; Krugman, 1995; Pollack, 1995). According to Krugman, narcissistic character pathology is "a caricature of the male gender role stereotype: emotionally unflappable, powerful, and in control" (p. 116).

The most often discussed cause of the above has been harsh gender role socialization (Levant, 1995; Kilmartin, 1991; Pleck, 1995; Pollack, 1995). However, harsh socialization of behavioral norms does not explain the origin of these norms. It does not explain the violence, misogyny, and emotional dissociation so characteristic of masculinity in so many cultures (Brooks & Silverstein, 1995). I have suggested that certain aspects of what we think of as "gendered" behavior for girls are largely an outcome of trauma and dissociation, and might be considered a "posttraumatic style." Much of stereotypical masculinity may also posttraumatic. While the key ingredients are still attachment and dissociation, as they are for girls, the trauma route is somewhat different for boys.

The sexual abuse of boys tend to be extrafamilial (79%-83%, prevalence figures from Lisak et al., 1996, and Finklehor, 1984, respectively) and out of the home. Sexually abused boys can develop dissociative symptoms, and highly dissociative boys may also have female gendered parts, resulting from identification with female aggressors and/or which execute the female linked tasks (Grand, 1997). While sexually abused boys can exhibit psychological patterns like those of girls, such as shame, depression, anxiety, suicidality, and self-mutilation, they are more likely than are sexually abused girls to behave aggressively toward others (Finkelhor, 1990; Gartner, 1999; Putnam, 1997). This is a complicated matter. A homophobic society in which needy vulnerability is equated with femininity–which is equated with homosexuality, especially does not foster integration of gender linked states in males.

Boys are subjected to very high levels of physical abuse. Perhaps because our culture teaches us that boys are supposed to be able to "take it," we don't always take in how serious this can be. Pollack (1998) cites a recent Navy study that found that 39% of its male recruits had been exposed to physical violence from their parents. A recent national survey of violent victimization of children and adolescents (Boney-McCoy & Finkelhor, 1995) found that about one half of the boys (47.4%) had been subjected to some form of violent victimization, including 18.4% who had been victims of aggravated assault, and 16.3% of simple assault. In addition, 13.5% had experienced genital violence–violence directed at the genitals with the intent of physical harm. Similarly, Pollack (1998) states that one in ten boys has been kicked in the groin before junior high school. At the same time that they are exposed to high levels of physical threat and violence, boys are socialized to experience and express anger (Fivush, 1989; Fuchs & Thelin, 1988; Kilmartin, 1991; Levant, 2000; Pleck, 1995) and discouraged from expressing emotional need and vulnerability (Unger & Crawford, 1995; Miller, 1976). In this way, a combination of childhood trauma, dissociation, and social pressure may push more boys in the direction of hypermasculinity and aggressivity.

In addition to physical and sexual abuse, boys are more often subjected to ruptures of attachment described as "the male wound" (Hudson & Jacot, 1991), and as a "normative developmental trauma" (Betcher & Pollack, 1993; Pollack, 1995; Pollack, 1998), both involving dissociation of affectional longings and resulting in fears of isolation and feelings of deprivation. Greenson (1968) coined the term "dis-identification" to refer to the (assumed) need for the *male* [emphasis added] child to emotionally separate himself from his primary object of identification, his mother. He felt that the boy then needed to "counter-identify" with the father in order to attain a healthy sense of masculinity. Hudson and Jacot (1991) refer to these two processes as "the male wound," a permanent psychical fissure or dissociation which generates difficulty with emotion. Stoller (1974, 1985) was even more specific stating that the boy must erect an internal "protective shield" of "symbiosis anxiety" against his early "protofemininity": "The first order of business in being a man is don't be a woman" (1985, p. 183). The achievement of masculine gender identity comes at the cost of repudiation of this identification with mother, and often, of everything that is female identified. Stoller's work, then, effectively turned Freud's viewpoint about the greater difficulty of the girl in attaining gender identity, on its head. Chodorow (1978), incorporating Stoller's observations into her earlier work on gender (1971, 1974), maintained that because women universally mother, the differences between the sexes will follow in accordance with their necessary identifications and disidentifications. Men, fearing merger and symbiosis, will have more rigid interpersonal ego boundaries, will be less relational and more patriarchal; and women, experiencing themselves and being experienced by their mothers as more like and connected each with the other, will be more relational. As did Stoller, Chodorow emphasized that masculinity comes to be defined as "not female."

It should be noted that Stoller's, and then Chodorow's, and then Gilligan's theorizing with regard to the above is based upon a Mahlerian (1975) concept of a symbiotic phase of development. Stern's (1985) seminal work on infant development casts much doubt upon the likelihood or extent of such a phase. In addition, recent anthropological theory, evidence, and reinterpretation of evidence (Eisler, 1987) suggests that despite probable near-universal mothering, not all cultures have been patriarchal. This, then, undermines the "protofemininity" perspective. Taken together, these cast some doubt on Chodorow's claim that near-universal mothering by women results in men who are less relational and more patriarchal. Perhaps the long-standing appeal of these theories has something to do with the unstated underlying femiphobic assumption that a boy's identification with mother and with femininity is to be feared, or is highly undesirable, at best. Herek (1987) has offered an interesting sociological explanation for the same construct–the belief that femininity taints masculinity and must therefore be avoided by "real" (heterosexual) men.

Pollack is the gender theorist who has most explicitly linked the masculine gendered style with trauma. He has postulated that, partly as a result of gender identity issues for the very young boy, "there may be a developmental basis for a gender-specific vulnerability to *traumatic abrogation* of the early holding environment . . . an *impingement* in boys' development–a normative life-cycle loss–that may, later in life, leave many adult men at risk for fears of intimate connection" (1995, p. 41). In his later work (1998), Pollack has suggested that the vulnerable period for boys is around the time they begin school and are pushed out of the nest by their mothers. His emphasis upon the potentially traumatogenic nature of this premature separation is consistent with a number of clinical and research findings suggestive of a common or frequent blunting or dissociation of emotional longings in men. He feels that one result of these repressed yearnings in males may be "the creation of *transitional* or *self-object* relationships with mother substitutes that are meant to repair and assuage the unspeakable hurt of premature traumatic separation and simultaneously to deny the loss of the relational bond" (1995, pp. 41-42).

In my view, Pollack's point that boys tend to be more vulnerable to premature separation from their mothers, and that some of the characteristics of male gendered behavior are derivative of traumatic separations, is an extremely important one. Here I would like to present a simpler alternative to the Stoller/Chodorow/Greenson/Hudson and Jacot perspective that the more rigid interpersonal ego boundaries, fears of merger and less relational characteristics associated with masculinity derive from the fact that the boy is a different gender from his early caretaking figure and must repudiate his identification with mother and females in order to achieve masculine gender identity. This alternative perspective is: perhaps the trauma of maternal emotional abandonment is, itself, genderless; but since this happens more often to boys, and since masculinity becomes narcissistically invested with "superiority," the privilege of being so deprived becomes cherished, as part of the gender role. This hypothesis is consistent with the cognitive developmental theory of gender typing (Kohlberg, 1966), according to which gender identity precedes and organizes gendered behaviors (i.e., "I am a boy; therefore I do boy things," "Boys don't cry or get sad; I get mad–because I am a boy"). As noted earlier, the often compensatory narcissistic patterns, in addition to the dissociation of emotional vulnerability and attachment need are also components of stereotypical "masculinity" (Krugman, 1995; Levant, 1995; Pollack, 1995). This "male pattern" is more characteristic of males, but not specific to them. There are clinical and anecdotal reports of girls who have cut off their attachment longings, who exhibit some of the same characteristics of blunted emotionality, ragefulness, and narcissism.

The Coriolanus Complex: The Warrior

One important variant of this masculine pattern might be called the Coriolanus complex. Coriolanus, a fifth century, BC Roman patrician, was the tragic hero of one of Shakespeare's lesser known plays. In *Coriolanus*, the play, Corialanus personifies the warrior mentality. He was close to his mother, but was banished from her presence as a young child so that he would become the kind of man that she admired–a fierce, emotionally illiterate warrior. The tragedy is in how his banishment from the possibility of needing his mother (a woman incapable of loving her little boy and who used him as her narcissistic extension, her warrior), deforms his humanity: his need for attachment is dissociated, he becomes brutally narcissistic, and his emotionality/rage redirected into war. And he is once again, as an adult, banished from his city that he needs and loves, because he had become so characterologically damaged. Stoller and Herdt (1985) offer a description of the Sambia, a New Guinea tribe, notable for its fierce warriors and its extreme devaluation and fear of femininity. The boys in this tribe spent their early childhood in extreme, perhaps "blissful" physical closeness to their mothers, only to be suddenly and forcibly ripped away, sometimes from their mothers' arms, to live in an all-male community. These men who were physically close, affectionate, and dependent upon their mothers and who were then traumatically separated from their mothers while still children, became fierce warriors, and misogynistic, heterosexual husbands. While Stoller and Herdt used this to support a specific argument, it also supports the more general one made here–that the premature, forced cut off of emotional longings can be traumatic, inducing a kind of blind rage that can be effectively redirected in war. And, males may be genetically predisposed to respond to trauma with aggressivity (Perry, 1999).

In sum, boys, like girls, are exposed to very high rates of trauma, including physical, sexual, and emotional abuse; but unlike girls, boys are often routinely deprived of one important means to deal with their trauma: emotional closeness with their mothers and/or other attachment figures. In particular, if they have blunted or cut off vulnerability and emotional neediness, which becomes part of their male gender role identity, they are limited in their ability to grieve, which is also necessary in resolving trauma and loss (Pleck, 1995). Thus, much of what appears normative gender may be posttraumatic. Perhaps it is not just socialization–learning, modeling, etc., but, importantly, also trauma, that contributes to the more problematic masculine attributes considered normative: the "give 'em Hell!" hyperaggressivity, the "no sissy stuff," and the narcissistic "big wheel."

Bruce Perry's Contribution to Evolutionary Theory

The last decade has seen remarkable progress in the understanding of the biological aspects of gender and gender identity (Breedlove, 1994; Colopinto, 1999; Diamond & Signumdson, 1997; Halpern, 1997; Hoyenga, 1993). Now we know much more than before about the undeniable impact of genes and hormones on much of sex-differentiated abilities and behavior. However, along with this has come a greater degree of sophistication such that the "either-or" model, or nature versus nurture, has generally been replaced with a psychobiosocial model in which determinism is understood to be highly interactive and in which specific, unitary causes are not always isolatable (Halpern, 1997; Schore, 1998).

Particularly exciting in this new wave of research-generated knowledge are Bruce Perry's (1999, 2000) findings with respect to the tendency of children's physiological responses to trauma to be sex-differentiated, suggesting differing biological predispositions for the form of posttraumatic physiological response. Perry describes how exposure to trauma affects neurodevelopmental processes: hyper- and hypoarousal responses become more pronounced with more early, severe, and chronic trauma. Perry found that while both sexes employ both kinds of responses, that boys' responses to trauma tend more toward hyperarousal than do girls', while girls and very young children exhibit hypoarousal, "dissociative" responses. The hyperarousal response involves "fight/flight," which begins as a neurophysiological alarm reaction and continues with elevated heart rate, startle response, behavioral irritability, and increased locomotion. The vigilance for threat can increase the probability of aggression. Hypoarousal involves dissociative symptoms such as fugue, numbing, fantasy, analgesia, derealization, depersonalization, catatonia, and fainting. This defeat response, characterized by robotic compliance, glazed expressions, passivity, and decreased heart rates, is similar to "learned helplessness." Perry postulates an evolutionary basis for his findings. In his "environment of evolutionary adaptiveness," men caught in an enemy attack were more likely to be killed, while the women and young children were more likely to be captured. Men's best chance of survival would be to attack or flee, while women's and young children's would be in the dissociative freeze response, which is adaptive to immobilization or inescapable pain.

Adding Perry's information to what we know about the socialization process can be helpful. In particular, it underscores how the posttraumatic aggressivity of boys may appear indistinguishable from stereotypical "masculinity," disguising the trauma and pain underneath. It also underscores how girls' posttraumatic responses are more often dissociative and apparently passive (the freeze response). Both aggressivity and passivity are considered aspects of stereotypical gender, and therefore prescriptive. It is probably more adaptive for us today, to see the heightened gendered form of these responses, not as prescriptive, but as posttraumatic–symptomatic of unresolved pain, trauma, and grief.

The Reproduction of Pathological Gender

Gender is reproduced in many ways. It is elicited by social context, learned, internalized, socially constructed, reenacted, and so on. For purposes of this paper, the primary emphasis is upon the reproduction of pathological gender via the cycle of abuse. While a number of studies have indicated that most perpetrators of violence and abuse were themselves abused (Finkelhor, 1990; Romano & de Luca, 1997), most victims do not go on to become perpetrators (Gartner, 1999; Lisak et al., 1966). Thus, the prevalence of abuse would decrease if it were not for the fact that perpetrators tend to have multiple victims and to be recidivists. One of the problems is the misreading of posttraumatic hyper-aggressivity and violence as normative, a "boys will be boys" point of view. Intertwined with this is the tendency for the descriptive to become prescriptive. In this way, observed male behavior becomes the way males *should* behave. This "is to ought" fallacy needs to be repeatedly addressed, and we need more interventions to help hyper-aggressive males deal with their emotions.

Another pathway is via projective identification and mutual projective identification, whereby individuals and dyads, respectively, may project affects and states that are least gender "appropriate" into and onto others, as well as into other parts of the self. For example, if a woman projects her rage into an already hyperaggressive male, this may not only be immediately dangerous to herself, but it perpetuates the traumatogenic culture both in herself and in the others involved. Or a male may project gender "inappropriate" feelings of neediness into other individuals whom he then physically punishes for what he has disavowed in himself. Such aggression, then, may be traumatic to the others involved, reproducing gendered states in them. In his book, *The Batterer*, Dutton (1995) introduces another perspective on the phenomenon of near-universal mothering: "One reality that may differentiate boys from girls is that the former develop a stronger bond to an opposite gender person at an earlier developmental stage." (p. 107). In adult heterosexual relationships, the man's attachment figure is female, like his mother. If the boy has been intermittently abused in the context of his early attachment or if his security needs have otherwise been overly frustrated, his attachment needs are likely to be intensified, and the threat of separation is likely to produce very strong responses–often very terrified and angry ones. While the anger may be motivated by a desire for soothing, its violent expression can be devastating. This configuration is an important one in the reproduction of gender, especially since children may be witnessing this parental, male-female violence.

An additional problem is the all too frequent collective and individual denial and unwillingness to do what it takes to ensure the cessation of the abuse of children. Most perpetrators are male. One effect of the patriarchal power structure is to give a covert license to abusive perpetrators of terror within our own culture. Since this confuses victims and bystanders, it gives added cover to perpetrators (Herman, 1981).

CONCLUSION

This article proposes that trauma contributes substantially to the creation of "gendered" states. With increasing psychological health and ability to grieve, these gendered states tend to become better integrated. It is my hope that the foregoing formulation–that much of the pathological gendered behavior (which is so endemic in our culture) has roots in trauma–may help us to better understand and reduce this kind of trauma in the future.

REFERENCES

Allport, G.W. (1954). *The nature of prejudice*. Cambridge, MA: Addison-Wesley.

Asher, S.J. (1988). The effects of childhood sexual abuse: A review of the issues and evidence. In L.E.A. Walker, (Ed.). *Handbook of sexual abuse of children*. New York: Springer Publishing Company.

Beauvoir, S. de (1953). *The second sex*. New York: Alfred A. Knopf.

Belenky, M.F., Clinchy, B.M., Goldberger, N.R., & Tarule, J.M. (1986). *Women's ways of knowing*. New York: Basic Books.

Bem, S.L. (1983). Gender schema theory and its implications for child development: Raising gender-aschematic children in a gender-schematic society. *Signs*, *8*, 367-389.

Benatar, M. (2000). A qualitative study of the effect of a history of childhood sexual abuse on therapists who treat survivors of sexual abuse. *Journal of Trauma and Dissociation*, *1*(3), 9-28.

Betcher, R.W., & Pollack, W.S. (1993). *In a time of fallen heroes*. New York: Guilford Press.

Blizard, R.A. (1997). The origins of dissociative identity disorder from an object relations theory and attachment theory perspective. *Dissociation*, *10*(4), 246-254.

Blizard, R.A. (2001). Masochistic and sadistic ego states: Dissociative solutions to the dilemma of attachment to an abusive caretaker. *Journal of Trauma and Dissociation*, *2*(4), 37-58.

Block, J.B (1984). *Sex role identity and ego development*. San Francisco: Josey Bass.

Block, J.H. (1973). Conceptions of sex role. *American Psychologist*, *28*, 512-526.

Bohan, J.S. (1993). Regarding gender: essentialism, constructionism, and feminist psychology. *Psychology of Women Quarterly*, *17*, 5-21.

Boney-McCoy, S., & Finkelhor, D. (1995). Psychosocial sequelae of violent victimization in a national youth sample. *Journal of Consulting and Clinical Psychology*, *63*, 726-736.

Boney-McCoy, S., & Finkelhor, D. (1996). Is youth victimization related to trauma symptoms and depression after controlling for prior symptoms and family relationships? A longitudinal, prospective study. *Journal of Consulting and Clinical Psychology, 64*, 1406-1416.

Braebeck, M.M. (Ed.). (1989). *Theory, research, and educational implications of the ethic of care*. New York: Praeger.

Brannon, R. (1976). The male sex role: Our culture's blueprint for manhood, what it's done for us lately. In D. David and R. Brannon (Eds.).*The forty-nine percept majority: The male sex role* (pp. 1-48). Reading, MA: Addison-Wesley.

Breedlove, S.M. (1994). Sexual differentiation of the human nervous system. *Annual Review of Psychology, 45*, 389-418.

Brooks, G.R., & Silverstein, L.B (1995). Understanding the dark side of masculinity: An interactive systems model. In R.F. Levant. & W.S. Pollack (Eds.), *A new psychology of men* (pp. 280-336). New York: Basic Books.

Brown, L.S. (1991). Not outside the range: One feminist perspective on psychic trauma. *American Imago, 48*, 119-133.

Brown, L.S. (1992). A feminist critique of the personality disorders. In L.S. Brown, & M. Ballou (Eds.), *Personality and psychopathology: Feminist reappraisals* (pp. 206-228). New York: Guilford.

Brown, L.M., & Gilligan, C. (1992). *Meeting at the crossroads*. New York: Ballantine Books.

Brownmiller, S. (1975). *Against our will: Men, women, and rape*. New York: Simon and Schuster.

Broverman, I.K., Broverman, D.M., Clarkson, F.E., Rosenkrantz, P.S., & Vogel, S.R. (1970). Sex-role stereotypes and clinical judgments of mental health. *Journal of Consulting and Clinical Psychology, 34*, 1-7.

Chodorow, N. (1971). "Being and doing": A cross cultural examination of the socialization of males and females. In V. Gornick and B.K. Moran (Eds.), *Women in sexist society: Studies in power and powerlessness* (pp. 173-197). New York: Basic Books.

Chodorow, N. (1974). Family structure and feminine personality. In M.Z. Rosaldo, & L. Lamphere (Eds.), *Woman, culture and society* (pp. 43-66). Stanford, CA: Stanford University Press.

Chodorow, N. (1978). *The reproduction of mothering*. Berkeley: University of California Press.

Chu, J.A. (1998). *Rebuilding shattered lives*. New York: John Wiley & Sons.

Chu, J.A. (2001). A decline in the abuse of children? *Journal of Trauma and Dissociation, 2*(2), 1-4.

Clopton, N., & Sorell, G. (1993). Gender differences in moral reasoning: Stable or situational? *Psychology of Women Quarterly, 17*, 85-101.

Coates, S.W., & Moore, M.S. (1997). The complexity of early trauma: Representation and transformation. *Psychoanalytic Inquiry, 17*, 286-311.

Colapinto, J. (2000). *As nature made him: The boy who was raised as a girl*. New York: Harper Collins.

Copjec, J. (1994). *Read my desire*. Cambridge, MA: MIT Press.

Danieli, Y. (1985). The treatment and prevention of long-term effects and intergenerational transmission of victimization: A lesson from holocaust survivors and their children. In C.R. Figley (Ed.), *The study and treatment of post-traumatic stress disorder* (pp. 295-313). New York: Bruner/Mazel.

Davies, J.M., & Frawley, M.G. (1994). *Treating the adult survivor of childhood sexual abuse*. New York: Basic Books.

Diamond, M., & Sigmundson, H. K. (1997). Sex reassignment at birth: A long term review and clinical implications. *Archives of Pediatric and Adolescent Medicine, 151*, 298-304.

Dinnerstein, D. (1976). *The mermaid and the Minotaur*. New York: Harper and Row.

Dutton, D.G., with Gollant, S.K. (1995). *The batterer: A psychological profile*. New York: Basic Books.

Dyess, C., & Dean, T. (2000). Gender: The impossibility of meaning. *Psychoanalytic Dialogues, 10*, 735-756.

Espin, O.M., & Gawelek, M.A. (1992). Women's diversity: Ethnicity, race, class, and gender in theories of feminist psychology. In L.S. Brown and M. Ballou (Eds.), *Personality and psychopathology: Feminist reappraisals* (pp. 88-108). New York: Guilford.

Ferenczi, S. (1949). Confusion of tongues between the adult and the child. *International Journal of Psycho-Analysis, 30*, 225-231.

Finkelhor, D. (1984). *Child sexual abuse: New theory and research*. New York: Free Press.

Finkelhor, D. (1990). Early and long term effects of child sexual abuse: an update. *Professional Psychology: Research and Practice, 21*, 325-330.

Finkelhor, D., & Dziuba-Leatherman, J. (1994). Victimization of children. *The American Psychologist, 49*, 173-183.

Fitzgerald, L.F. (1993). Sexual harassment: Violence against women in the workplace. *American Psychologist, 48*, 1070-1076.

Fivush, R. (1989). Exploring sex differences in the emotional content of mother-child conversations about the past. *Sex Roles, 20*, 675-691.

Freyd, J.J. (1996). *Betrayal trauma: The logic of forgetting childhood abuse*. Cambridge, MA: Harvard University Press.

Friedan, B. (1963). *The feminine mystique*. New York: Dell.

Fuchs, D., & Thelen, M.H. (1988). Children's expected interpersonal consequences of communicating their affective state and reported likelihood of expression. *Child Development, 59*, 1314-1322.

Gartner, R.B. (1999). *Betrayed as boys*. New York: Basic Books.

Giddings, P. (1984). *When and where I enter: The impact of black women on race and sex in America*. New York: Bantam.

Gilligan, C. (1982). *In a different voice*. Cambridge, MA: Harvard University Press.

Gilligan, C., & Attanuccu, J. (1988). Two moral orientations. In C. Gilligan, C. J. Ward, & J. M. Taylor, with B. Bartage (Eds.), *Mapping the moral domain: A contribution of women's thinking to psychological theory and education* (pp. 73-86). Cambridge, MA: Harvard University Press.

Grand, S. (1997). On the gendering of traumatic dissociation: A case of mother-son incest. *Gender and Psychoanalysis, 1*, 55-77.

Greenson, R.R. (1968). Dis-identifying from mother: Its special importance for the boy. *International Journal of Psycho-analysis, 49*, 370.

Hacker, H.M. (1981). Women as a minority group. In Cox, S. (Ed.), *Female psychology: The emerging self* (pp. 164-178). New York: St. Martin's Press.

Halpern, D.F. (1997). Sex differences in intelligence: implications for education. *American Psychologist, 52*, 1091-1102.

Hare-Mustin, R.T., & Marecek, J. (1988). The meaning of difference: gender theory, postmodernism, and psychology. *American Psychologist, 43*, 455-462.

Hare-Mustin, R.T., & Marecek, J. (1990). Gender and the meaning of difference: Postmodernism and psychology. In R.T. Hare-Mustin, & J. Marecek (Eds.), *Making a difference: Psychology and the construction of gender* (pp. 22-64). New Haven: Yale University Press.

Herek, G.M. (1987). On heterosexual masculinity: Some psychical consequences of the social construction of gender and sexual orientation. In M.S. Kimmel (Ed.), *Changing men: New directions in research on men and masculinity* (pp. 68-82). Newbury Park, CA: Sage Press.

Herman, J.L., with Hirschman, L. (1981). *Father-daughter incest.* Cambridge, MA: Harvard University Press.

Herman, J.L. (1992). *Trauma and recovery.* New York: Basic Books.

Hooks, B. (1984). *Feminist theory: From margin to center.* Boston: South End Press.

Hooks, B. (1989). *Talking back: Thinking feminist, thinking black.* Boston: South End Press.

Horney, K. (1934). The overvaluation of love. *Psychoanalytic Quarterly, III*, 605-638.

Howell, E.F. (1975). Self presentation in reference to sex role stereotypes as related to level of moral development. Unpublished doctoral dissertation. New York University.

Howell, E.F. (1981). Women: from Freud to the present. In E. Howell, & M. Bayes, (Eds.) *Women and mental health* (pp. 3-25). New York: Basic Books.

Howell, E.F. (in press). Back to the "states": Victim and abuser states in borderline personality disorder. *Psychoanalytic Dialogues.*

Hoyenga, K.B., & Hoyenga, K.T. (1993). *Gender-related differences.* Needham Heights, MA: Allyn and Bacon.

Hudson, L., & Jacot, B. (1991). *The way men think: Intellect, intimacy, and the erotic imagination.* New Haven: Yale University Press.

Hurtado, A. (1989). Relating to privilege: Seduction and rejection in the subordination of white women and women of color. *Signs: Journal of Women in Culture and Society, 14*, 833-855.

Jordan, J.V., Kaplan, A.G., Miller, J.B., Stiver, I.P., & Surry, J.L. (1991). *Women's growth in connection.* New York: Guilford Press.

Kemelgor, C., & Etzowitz, H. (2001). Overcoming isolation: women's dilemmas in American academic sciences. *Minerva, 39*, 239-257.

Kilmartin, C.T. (1994). *The masculine self.* New York: MacMillan Press.

Kohlberg, L. (1966). A cognitive-development analysis of children's sex-role concepts and attitudes. In E.E. Maccoby (Ed.), *The development of sex differences* (pp. 82-173). Stanford, CA: Stanford University Press.

Koss, M.P. (1993). Rape: Scope, impact, interventions and public policy responses. *American Psychologist, 48*, 1062-1069.

Krugman, S. (1995). Male development and the transformation of shame. In R.F. Levant, & W.S. Pollack (Eds.), *A new psychology of men*. New York: Basic Books.

Landrine, H. (1989). The politics of personality disorder. *Psychology of Women Quarterly, 13*, 325-339.

Layton, L. (1998). *Who's that girl? Who's that boy? Clinical practice meets postmodern gender theory*. Northvale, NJ: Jason Aronson.

Lerman, H. (1986). From Freud to feminist personality theory: Getting there from here. *Psychology of Women Quarterly, 7*, 313-328.

Lerner, H.E. (1982). Special issues of women in psychotherapy. In M.T. Notman and C.C. Nadelson (Eds.), *The woman patient, Vol. 3: Aggression, adaptations, and psychotherapy* (pp. 273-286). New York: Plenum Press.

Levant, R.F. (1995). Toward a reconstruction of masculinity. In R.F. Levant, & W.S. Pollack (Eds.), *A new psychology of men* (pp. 229-251). New York: Basic Books.

Little, L., & Hamby, S.L. (1999). *Professional Psychology: Research and Practice*. 30:4, 378-385.

Lisak, D., Hopper, J., & Song, P. (1996). Factors in the cycle of violence: Gender rigidity and emotional constriction. *Journal of Traumatic Stress, 4*, 721-743.

Lott, B. (1990). Dual natures or learned behaviors? In R.T. Hare-Mustin, & J. Marecek (Eds.), *Making a difference: Psychology and the construction of gender* (pp. 65-101). New Haven: Yale University Press.

Maccoby, E.E. (1966). Sex differences in intellectual functioning. In. E.E. Maccoby, *The development of sex differences* (pp. 25-55). Stanford, CA: Stanford University Press.

Maccoby, E.E. (1990). Gender and relationships: A developmental account. *American Psychologist, 45*, 513-520.

Mahler, M.S., Pine, F., & Bergman, A. (1975). *The psychological birth of the human infant*. New York: Basic Books.

Mednick, M.T. (1989). On the politics of psychological constructs: Stop the bandwagon, I want to get off. *American Psychologist, 44*, 1118-1123.

Mill, J.S. (1972/1869). The subjection of women. In M. Schneir (Ed.), *Feminism: The essential historical writings* (pp. 162-178). New York: Vintage.

Miller, J.B. (1976). *Toward a new psychology of women*. Boston: Beacon Press.

Nijenhuis, E.R.S., Spinhoven P., van Dyck, R., & van der Hart, O. (1998). Degree of somatoform and psychological dissociation in dissociative disorder is correlated with reported trauma. *Journal of Traumatic Stress, 11*, 711-730.

Nijenhuis, E.R.S., Vanderlinden, J., & Spinhoven, P. (1998). Animal defensive reactions as a model for trauma-induced dissociative reaction. *Journal of Traumatic Stress, 11*, 243-260.

Perry, B.D. (1999). Neurodevelopment and dissociation: Trauma and adaptive responses to fear. Plenary paper presented at the 17th International Fall Conference of the International Society for the Study of Dissociation, November 14, 2000.

Perry, B.D. (2000). The memories of states: How the brain stores and retrieves traumatic experience. In Goodwin, J.M., & R.A. Attias, (Eds.), *Images of the body in trauma* (pp. 9-38). New York: Basic Books.

Pinker, S. (1994). *The language instinct.* New York: Harper Collins.

Pleck, J.H. (1995). The gender role strain paradigm: an update. In R.F. Levant, & W.S. Pollack (Eds.), *A new psychology of men*, (pp. 11-32). New York: Basic Books.

Pollack, W.S. (1995). No man is an island: a new psychoanalytic psychology of men. In R.F. Levant, & W.S. Pollack (Eds.), *A new psychology of men* (pp. 33-67). New York: Basic Books.

Pollack, W.S. (1998). *Real boys.* New York: Random House.

Profitt, N.J. (2000). *Psychological trauma, and the politics of resistance.* Binghamton, NY: The Haworth Press, Inc.

Putnam, F.W. (1997). *Dissociation in children and adolescents.* New York: Guilford Press.

Raine, N.V. (1998). *After silence: Rape and my journey back.* New York: Crown Publishers.

Rivera, M. (1989). Linking the psychological and the social: feminism, poststructuralism and multiple personality. *Dissociation*, *2*(1), 24-31.

Rivera, M. (1988). Am I a boy or girl? Multiple personality as a window on gender differences. *Resources for Feminist Research/Documentation sur la recherche féministe*, *17*(2), 41-45.

Romano. E., & de Luca, R.V. (1997). Exploring the relationship between childhood sexual abuse and adult sexual perpetration. *Journal of Family Violence*, *12*(1), 85-98.

Root, M.P. (1992). Reconstructing the impact of trauma on personality. In L.S. Brown and M. Ballou (Eds.), *Personality and psychopathology: Feminist reappraisals* (pp. 229-265). New York: Guilford.

Russell, D.E.H. (1986). *The secret trauma: Incest in the lives of girls and women.* New York: Basic Books.

Schafer, R. (1974). Problems in Freud's psychology of women. *Journal of the American Psychoanalytic Association*, *22*, 459-485.

Schetky, D.H. (1990). A review of the literature on the long-term effects of childhood sexual abuse. In R.P. Kluft (Ed.), *Incest-related syndromes of adult psychopathology* (pp. 35-54). Washington, DC: American Psychiatric Press.

Schore, A.N. (1997). *Affect regulation and the origin of the self.* New York: Lawrence Erlbaum Publishers.

Shainess, N. (1970). A psychiatrist's view: Images of women–past and present, overt and obscured. In R. Morgan, (Ed.), *Sisterhood is powerful: An anthology of writings from the women's liberation movement* (pp. 230-244). New York: Vintage Books.

Shusta, S.R. (1999). Successful treatment of refractory obsessive-compulsive disorder. *American Journal of Psychotherapy*, *53*, 372-391.

Spiegel, D. (1990). Trauma, dissociation, and hypnosis. In R.P. Kluft (Ed.), *Incest-related syndromes of adult psychopathology* (pp. 247-262). Washington, DC: American Psychiatric Press.

Stern, D. (1985). *The interpersonal world of the infant.* New York: Basic Books.

Stern, D.B. (2000). The limits of social construction: Commentary on paper by Cynthia Dyess and Tim Dean. *Psychoanalytic Dialogues*, *10*, 757-769.

Stoller, R.J. (1974). Symbiosis anxiety–The development of masculinity. *Archives of General Psychiatry*, *30*, 164-172.

Stoller, R.J. (1985). *Presentations of gender*. New Haven, CT: Yale University Press.

Stoller, R.J., & Herdt, G. (1985). The development of masculinity: A cross-cultural contribution. In R. Stoller (Ed.), *Presentations of gender* (pp. 181-199). New Haven, CT: Yale University Press.

Thompson, C. (1942). Cultural pressures in the psychology of women. *Psychiatry*, *5*, 331-339.

Unger, R.K. (1990). Imperfect reflections of reality: Psychology constructs gender. In R. Hare-Mustin, & J. Marecek (Eds.), *Making a difference: Psychology and the construction of gender* (pp. 102-149). New Haven, CT: Yale University Press.

Unger, R.K., & Crawford, M. (1992). *Women and gender: A feminist psychology*. New York: McGraw Hill.

Waites, E.A. (1993). *Trauma and survival: post-traumatic and dissociative disorders in women*4. New York: Norton.

Informed and Supportive Treatment for Lesbian, Gay, Bisexual and Transgendered Trauma Survivors

Margo Rivera, PhD

SUMMARY. It is widely acknowledged that sexuality is often a key area of conflict for individuals who have been traumatized and exploited in childhood. Most treatment regimens for trauma survivors include some focus on enhancing client's capacity to create a healthy adult sexuality, with the goal of replacing rigid, maladaptive beliefs and behaviors, rooted in childhood patterns of oppressive sexuality, with those that enable them to develop a mature and satisfying life. However, though sexuality is emphasized as a significant aspect of human functioning and one in which a traumatized individual frequently needs help, there is often little acknowledgement that there are a range of healthy expressions of sexuality and gender. Though most clients and most therapists are het-

---

Margo Rivera is affiliated with the Department of Psychiatry, Queen's University, Kingston, Ontario, Canada.

Address correspondence to: Margo Rivera, PhD, PCCC–Mental Health Services, Postal Bag 603, 752 King Street West, Kingston, ON K7L 4X3, Canada (E-mail: riveram@pccc.kari.net).

Some sections of this article were adapted from Rivera, M. (1996). *More alike than different: Treatment of severely dissociative trauma survivors*. Toronto: University of Toronto Press; and Rivera, M., & Wachob, S. (in press). Treatment of gay, lesbian, bisexual, and transgender survivors of child sexual abuse. In L.E.A. Walker, S.W. Gold, & B.A. Lucenko (Eds.), *Handbook on sexual abuse of children: Assessment, treatment & legal issues*. New York: Springer.

[Haworth co-indexing entry note]: "Informed and Supportive Treatment for Lesbian, Gay, Bisexual and Transgendered Trauma Survivors." Rivera, Margo. Co-published simultaneously in *Journal of Trauma & Dissociation* (The Haworth Medical Press, an imprint of The Haworth Press, Inc.) Vol. 3, No. 4, 2002, pp. 33-58; and: *Trauma and Sexuality: The Effects of Childhood Sexual, Physical, and Emotional Abuse on Sexuality Identity and Behavior* (ed: James A. Chu, and Elizabeth S. Bowman) The Haworth Medical Press, an imprint of The Haworth Press, Inc., 2002, pp. 33-58. Single or multiple copies of this article are available for a fee from The Haworth Document Delivery Service [1-800-HAWORTH, 9:00 a.m. - 5:00 p.m. (EST). E-mail address: getinfo@haworthpressinc.com].

erosexual, those clients who do not fit the norm in this regard need a therapeutic context in which their expressions of gender identity and sexual orientation are acknowledged and clearly supported, so that their psychotherapy process will enable them to learn to live freely and fully, rather than reinforcing the marginalization they experienced as abused children and as adults who practice sexualities which are not widely accepted and fully supported in our society.

KEYWORDS. Gay, lesbian, bisexual, transgender psychotherapy

INTRODUCTION

Most individuals who suffer from severe dissociative disorders report childhood histories of sexual abuse and exploitation. They tend to have many distorted and self-destructive beliefs about sexuality and particularly their own sexuality. As children and adolescents, they have often known sex as enforced or manipulated, as shameful and secretive, and they are unlikely to perceive their adult sexuality as a positive expression of their most authentic selves.

Similarly, many lesbians, gay men, bisexuals, and transgendered individuals (LGBT), whose experience of gender and sexual desire is all too often labeled "abnormal," meaning not only different but bad, must struggle with both external and internal prejudice. People with histories of sexual exploitation tend to be particularly vulnerable to the psychological effects of living in a climate of pervasive homophobia. The challenge of being lesbian, gay, bisexual, or transgendered is difficult enough to manage for someone who has not been traumatized in childhood. That challenge is exponentially increased when the individual is also struggling with a history of sexual abuse.

Psychotherapists who treat LGBT trauma survivors must be prepared to address both aspects of our clients' struggles. This article will examine some issues of relevance to mental health professionals who treat trauma survivors with the goal of enabling us to engage in an informed and constructive therapeutic dialogue that will lead to greater satisfaction with treatment and improved quality of care for our lesbian, gay, bisexual, and transgendered clients.

HETEROSEXISM AND TREATMENT PROFESSIONALS

"No problem. I can treat anyone. Human beings are all alike, and I am not prejudiced."

It is not uncommon for mental health professionals to discount the notion that we might be limited in our capacity to understand the struggles of our clients who are not heterosexual. Whether we have had any training in working with lesbian, gay, bisexual, and transgendered clients or not, few clinicians consider that treating such clients might be outside our area of competence (American Psychological Association, 1991; Clark & Serovich, 1997; Garnets & Kimmel, 1991; Hancock, 1995). Therapists frequently declare that people are people, and what they do in their bedrooms is their own business. It is important in this, and other areas, that we question the assumption that our education, training, and life experience as middle-class professionals necessarily equips us to offer informed treatment to anyone of any race, class, culture, or sexual orientation.

We may be guilty of a sort of selective blindness regarding experiences not our own, including the particular experience of the lesbian, gay, bisexual, or transgendered client. Mental health professionals are no less likely than anyone else to be socialized in our formative years to conventional and unexamined beliefs about sexuality. Even if we are not obviously homophobic, we are unlikely to be free from heterosexism–that worldview that assumes heterosexuality to be the standard against which every other form of gender and sexual expression is measured. Such is the degree of pervasive heterosexism in our culture that even therapists who are not themselves heterosexual may sometimes deny, denigrate, or stigmatize non-heterosexual forms of behavior, identity, relationship, or community. This can result in the devaluation of vital aspects of the lesbian, gay, bisexual, or transgendered client's life and healthy, functional relationships within the client's sexual and gender communities (Group for the Advancement of Psychiatry, 2000).

The difficulty is not that therapists are particularly prejudiced. With a few atavistic exceptions, the majority of mental health service providers exhibit much lower levels of homophobia than the general public (Breschke & Matthers, 1996; Gelso, Fassinger, Gomez, & Latts, 1995; Hayes & Gelso, 1993). However, many practitioners, despite a general willingness to be supportive of their lesbian, gay, bisexual, and transgendered clients' sexual and gender identities, are both vulnerable to acting on the basis of stereotypes (Garnets & Kimmel, 1991; Gelso et al., 1995; Hayes & Gelso, 1993) and not aware of the unique issues confronting the LGBT client (Buhrke & Douce, 1991; McHenry & Johnson, 1993; Morrow, 2000).

There is very little education in professional training programs about the experiences of lesbian, gay, bisexual, or transgendered individuals that would be likely to challenge, enrich, or offer some balance to the pervasive heterosexist values we learn as children and which are reinforced every day of our lives as adults. Therapists' prejudices and myopia are, therefore, rarely uncovered in our training. They can easily go unnoticed and then be enacted in ways that are harmful to our clients. This can lead to pathologizing aspects of the client's functioning, simply because certain beliefs and practices that are deeply meaningful to a client are not familiar or are anxiety-provoking to the therapist.

Without specialized continuing education and consultation, therapists may ignore central concerns in the lesbian, gay, bisexual, or transgendered individual's life. We may not be able to help our clients with the daunting challenges of living in a homophobic environment that continually assaults the sense of self. We may not be able to support our LGBT clients in creating self-affirming identities, satisfying relationships of which they can be proud, and active supportive communities (Brown, 1995). The result can be clients who terminate therapy as oppressed–or even more so–than when they began.

A more pervasive, and possibly less obvious, consequence of a heterosexist viewpoint is the limitations it places on the capacity to create an empathic therapeutic relationship. Empathy–the therapist's ability to allow another individual's experience to resonate within, such that it can be processed from a similar vantage point–is a basic tool of the psychotherapy process. When the therapeutic relationship is one in which the client can count on the therapist to provide an atmosphere of steady empathic connection, only occasionally ruptured with significant misunderstanding, this can provide a powerful healing matrix. Most persons' sense of self is enhanced by the awareness that someone else is focusing on them with a high degree of absorption, accurately understands their inner experience, and is responding with acceptance. Even when challenges to the person's thinking or behavior are offered, the empathic basis of the relationship offers the client the assurance that the self and the relationship are being enhanced rather than destroyed by such confrontations. Over time this empathic connection creates a milieu in which profound personal transformation can take place (Rivera, 1996). Any significant limitation on the therapist's capacity to develop the empathic aspect of the therapeutic relationship radically curtails the degree to which the client can grow and change within that context.

One of the ways in which mental health professionals can increase the likelihood of understanding the experiences of their lesbian, gay, bisexual, and transgendered clients is to familiarize themselves with the growing literature that addresses particular issues that may arise over the course of treatment. There is now a range of such resources. Until twenty-five years ago, almost all professional discussion of the issue assumed that "homosexuality"–as all LGBT behavior was invariably labeled–was a sign of profound psychopathology (Bergler, 1956; Caprio, 1954; Ellis, 1965; Socarides, 1968). These articles were mostly theoretical in nature, and the few empirical studies involved participants from hospitals or prisons (Moses & Hawkins, 1982). Kinsey and his colleagues (Kinsey, Pomeroy, & Martin, 1948; Kinsey, Pomeroy, Martin, & Gebhard, 1953) provided the earliest empirical data demonstrating that more people experience same-sex attraction, fantasy, and activity than had previously been believed. A few years later Hooker (1957) found no appreciable differences in the response profiles of thirty-five heterosexual men and thirty-five gay men to the Rorschach and the Thematic Apperception Test. This landmark study was the first of many to refute the prevailing assumption that same-sex orientations are pathological (Bieschke, McClanahan, Tozer, Grzegorek, & Park 2000).

Though a few mental health professionals still believe that same-sex or bisexual orientations are symptoms of mental illness, they are decidedly now the exception. In 1973, the category of homosexuality was removed as a mental disorder from the Diagnostic and Statistical Manual of the American Psychiatric Association, and gays, lesbians, and bisexuals were no longer officially deemed, by virtue of their sexual orientation, to have a mental disorder. In the past twenty years, popular and medical attributions of homosexuality as deviant have been thoroughly refuted, and there is now a body of social science literature that makes it clear that lesbians, gays, and bisexuals are no more likely to have psychological problems than anyone else (Lewis, 1980; Gottman, 1989; Green & Bozett, 1991). A careful review of the scientific literature indicates that there is no demonstrable relationship between sexual orientation and psychopathology (Gottman, 1989; Green & Bozett, 1991; Hooker, 1953; Hopkins, 1969; Lewis, 1980; Thompson, McCandless, & Strickland, 1971). Lesbian, gay, and bisexual clients seek treatment for the same reasons heterosexual clients do–Axis I & II psychiatric disorders and day-to-day stress, leading to decreased quality of life, suffering, and disability (Group for the Advancement of Psychiatry, 2000).

The mental health profession has not yet amassed research sufficient to decide the question of whether the transgendered person's experience of gender identity may be–like the orientations of lesbian, gay, and bisexual people–a normal variant, or whether it is a form of psychopathology, as is frequently assumed. The only two studies addressing the issue have found no empirical documentation for the general understanding that gender dysphoric individuals are severely pathological. An American study (Cole, O'Boyle, Emery, & Meyer, 1997) examined co-morbidity between gender dysphoria and psychopathology in 435 individuals. They found less than 10% evidenced problems associated with mental illness and suicide attempts. A subgroup completing the MMPI (N = 137) demonstrated profiles that were largely free of psychopathology, except that the Mf scales were more normal for the desired sex than the anatomical sex. A Norwegian study (Haralsen & Dahl, 2000) compared transsexuals (N = 86), personality disorder patients (N = 98), and healthy adult controls (N = 1068) on the SLC-90. They found that transsexuals scored significantly lower than personality disorder patients on all measures of psychopathology, and although the transsexuals generally scored slightly higher than the controls, their scores were well within normal limits. This is an area where more research is needed, but in any case, the transgendered person is likely to be on the receiving end of many of the same social prejudices (and, indeed, a few additional ones) that plague the lives of many lesbian, gay, and bisexual people and that result in a great deal of debilitating stress.

Many clinical books and articles have been published that present a positive view of lesbians, gays, and bisexuals, as well as direction for counseling them in evolving a healthy sexuality and a happy productive life (for example, D'Angelli & Patterson, 1995; Garnets & Kimmel, 1993; Gonsiorek & Weinrich, 1991; Perez, DeBord & Bieschke, 2000; American Psychological Association Guidelines for Treating Lesbian, Gay and Bisexual Clients, www.apa.org). There is very little social science literature that addresses the needs of transgendered clients, but mental health professionals should read with discrimination what there is (for example, Benjamin, 1966; Benjamin, 2001; Brown & Rounsley, 1996; Israel & Tarver, 1996) plus some literature from other fields (for example, Devor, 1997; Fineberg, 1993, 1996; Griggs, 1998), so as to increase our capacity to respond with accurate empathy to our transgendered clients.

An understanding of the particular issues facing lesbian, gay, bisexual, and transgendered clients can enable the psychotherapist to make a helpful assessment of an individual's difficulties and an effective plan for resolving them. Being aware of the pressures that LGBT individuals experience living as a sexual or gender minority in a homophobic and transphobic world, the informed practitioner can differentiate emotional disturbance that is largely reactive to present-day stresses from Axis I psychiatric illness. Axis II symptomatology, in which deep characterological problems may well be combined with difficulties adjusting to life as one of a sexual and/or gender minority, can be diagnosed without ignoring either the character pathology or the genuine life stresses that exacerbate personality problems. A sensitive and thorough assessment of this sort makes a planned therapeutic intervention much more likely to lead to deep, lasting, and positive psychosocial change, rather than diminishment and damage.

LESBIAN, GAY, BISEXUAL, TRANSGENDERED–NOT ALL THE SAME

Lesbians and gay men have sexual minority status in common, but their socialization as gendered beings, as women and men respectively, usually results in the development of a significantly different set of values and beliefs. (Brown, 1995; Downey & Friedman, 1995; Roth, 1985) Lesbians' socialization as women is likely to condition them to connect sex with love and commitment, thus the many jokes about what lesbians do on the second date ("hire a moving van"). The privileging of sex for its own sake is more rarely a value among lesbians, in contrast to gay men, though, of course, there are many exceptions to such generalizations.

Sexually abused lesbians, socialized as women to be the nurturer in relationships, are likely to feel pressured to engage in sexual activity that makes them uncomfortable because they believe that is their responsibility to meet their partners' needs, rather than because they must live up to an image of themselves as sexually avid and skilled lovers (as some gay may need to do). When, often as part of a recovery process, the lesbian comes to understand that meeting another's needs at the expense of your own is neither necessary nor necessarily truly caring, she is much more likely to abstain from sexual expression altogether, without much awareness of the toll such abstinence can take on an intimate relationship if her partner still wants to have sex. Such all or nothing thinking–"I have to have sex no matter when or how anyone demands it," "I do not like sex," and "I will never have sex again"–is not uncommon in women whose sexuality is still powerfully tied up with early abuse experiences and is therefore more childlike than adult. Helping the lesbian abuse survivor develop a set of beliefs about herself that are more complex and adaptive to her present-day life, to replace the dichotomous ones learned in an oppressive childhood, is often part of an effective therapy process.

A primary definition of the gay man, both within the gay community and in the wider society, is through his sexuality–the presumption of intense and pervasive sexual interest and constant availability (Troiden, 1989; Green, 1996). For some survivors of child sexual abuse, who may experience sex as a reenactment of their childhood abuse, this focus may serve to reinforce deeply-held beliefs that are painful, shaming, and isolating. This may occur in a variety of ways, depending on the individual and how he incorporates and lives out his life experiences, past and present. Some gay male sexual abuse survivors, like any other survivors of childhood sexual abuse, are frightened by sexual activity. Not only do they not center their lives in a positive way around the expression of their sexuality, they may be afraid to touch and be touched and afraid even to talk about their fears. This difference can lead them to experience themselves as outsiders in the gay community, just as they felt like outsiders, different, and silenced throughout their childhood. Other gay male abuse survivors engage in compulsive and indiscriminate sex, despite getting little satisfaction from their experiences, believing that presenting themselves as objects for the use of others is the only way they can create the human connections they long for. This dynamic sometimes leads to exacerbated self-hatred and hopelessness about building lives in which sexual relationships can be based on mutual respect and love.

In the gay male community, a youthful appearance (adolescent body, smooth skin, slight build) is frequently privileged. Pornographic/erotic images are often accepted as an aid to sexual expression and may portray young men involved in a range of sexual activities. These images can be powerfully triggering for the gay male abuse survivor. What his peers find erotic, titillating, or even funny, may retraumatize him. An effective therapy with an individual who has difficulties identifying positively with other gay men because of his childhood abuse eventually helps him separate his experience of abusive sex as a child from his adult sexual relationships. This can make all the difference in his ability to develop a mature and satisfying sexual life. This does not mean that he has to conform to anyone else's values regarding sexuality–he may be an anti-pornography activist if he so chooses. But he can create his own beliefs from the position of a thoughtful adult, rather than from the reactivity of a helpless child.

Individuals who experience themselves as bisexual challenge the binary frameworks that characterize our conceptualizations about the diversity of human sexuality. In fact, monosexuality is probably a derivative of a primary bisexual or ambisexual plasticity in the human species. It is most likely our socialization, rather than a biological imperative, that makes us proponents of monosexuality (whether heterosexual or homosexual) as normative. Theorists and researchers from Freud onward have demonstrated that the boundaries between sexualities are quite fluid and that many more people than those who label themselves bisexual manage to experience multiple forms of sexual expression with partners of both sexes despite cultural dictates and institutional arrangements (Kinsey et al., 1948, 1953; Bell & Weinberg, 1978). In fact, Kinsey and his colleagues suggested that bisexuality may be more prevalent than homosexuality and encouraged researchers to think of sexuality in terms of a continuum, rather than as a set of dichotomous categories. Subsequent research has supported this notion of the fluid nature of sexual orientation (Blumstein & Schwartz, 1977; Klein and Wolf, 1985). However, despite this reality, there is little room for the ambisexual in our cultural, and sexual abuse survivors who experience themselves as bisexual may be seen as simply afraid to come out as lesbian or gay and may be pressured by peers to "get off the fence." Disapproval of bisexuality is particularly prevalent in the context of HIV/AIDS. Individuals who have sex with both men and women are often blamed for the transmission of the disease to "innocent victims," as if certain groups are especially entitled to immunity from this disease. Bisexual men are charged with spreading AIDS to their heterosexual female partners, and bisexual women are seen as importing AIDS into the lesbian community (Weinberg, Williams, & Pryor, 1994; Namaste, 1998), thus indicting bisexual orientation rather than an individual's dishonesty about multiple sexual partners and/or irresponsibility about safe sex, behaviors that are practiced by people of all sexual orientations.

Our society has been rigid in maintaining a two-gender system, to the exclusion of social and biological variations. However, some people with male biology grow up experiencing themselves as female; some with female biology as male. Others experience themselves as a blend of both male and female (androgynous), and still others experience themselves as neither male nor female but as an unidentified third gender or no gender at all (Cope & Darke, 1999). The term "transgender" has only recently come into popular use and includes all people whose felt sense of core gender identity does not correspond to their assigned sex at birth (MacDonald, 1998). People who are not able to fit into the binary gender categories (male/female) that we take for granted self-identify in a variety of ways. The term "transgendered" is used to describe a range of people who cross socially constructed gender boundaries. In this article, "transgendered man" and "transgendered woman" refer to the identity claimed by the individual, regardless of their sex assignment at birth or their status as pre, post, or non-operative transsexuals.

Transgendered women and men present even greater challenges to the way in which we invent categories, pigeonhole people, and try to force them to conform to our socially constructed expectations. The question of sex and the question of gender, though inextricably bound with each other, are not the same question (Rubin, 1984). Unfortunately, any distinction is all but erased in the public mind where effeminacy is often conflated with the identity of gay men and masculinity with that of lesbians. In fact, the most intense prejudices directed toward non-heterosexual individuals focus on their refusal to conform to gender stereotypes rather than the manner of their sexual expression. Drag queens, effeminate men, and butch women are the targets of the most vicious attacks from gay-bashers determined to beat them into submission to the gender codes our culture endorses. Not all transgendered individuals are lesbian or gay, but their inability or unwillingness to conform to our social imperatives about what women and men should look and act like links them with others who transgress social dictates about gender and sexuality.

CHILDHOOD SEXUAL TRAUMA AND HOMO/TRANSPHOBIA

Many adolescent and adult survivors of childhood trauma, especially those who have developed severe dissociative conditions, have experienced a range of traumas, including child sexual abuse (Putman, Guroff, Silberman, Barban, & Post, 1986; Ross Norton, & Wozney, 1989). It is developmentally normal for children to understand themselves as the source of all their experiences. They cannot understand the concept of random assignment of good fortune or ill treatment. They are assaulted and exploited because of who they are. Abused children are convinced that they must not let anyone know about what goes on in their lives because, though everyone can see that they are different, the best that they can hope for is that no one sees just how strange and how pernicious they are.

Similarly, lesbians, gay men, bisexuals, and transgendered people frequently struggle with internalized homophobia, fear and hatred of oneself as a sexual being with same-sex desires and affectional preferences, and/or internalized transphobia, fear and hatred of oneself as a person whose sense of gender identity does not match one's body. These are understandable responses to coming up repeatedly against the hatred and fear of any sexuality and gender identity that does not conform rigidly to cultural norms. Lesbian, gay, bisexual, and transgendered adults who were sexually exploited, assaulted, and oppressed as children find their experiences of being singled out, made to feel different, and hated and hurt by people in authority, and often by peers as well, replicated and perpetuated in adolescence and adulthood.

No matter which comes first, the abuse that entails some kind of attack on the body or the abuse that entails an attack on the sexual and/or gender identity of the person, the effect can be similar. Minimizing the effects of such attacks on one's self is critical. Unable to change the external world, the child, and later the adult, must develop ways to cushion the internal effects. There are a number of ways to accomplish this–dissociation, fantasy, drugs or alcohol, self-injury, use of food, sex, exercise, work, computers or any other substance or activity in a way that alters one's physical and or psychological chemistry. The problem with these methods is that they work well–temporarily. When children who have been sexually abused begins to notice their same-sex sexual attractions, or the children who have been scapegoated from very young because they do not conform to gender norms are then sexually assaulted, defenses that have worked to ameliorate the first painful reality are ready-made for this new situation. The therapist must be able to recognize the reality of both oppressions to help such an individual face and deal with each as it is reinforced by the other (Rivera & Wachob, in press).

ORIGINS OF SEXUAL ORIENTATION AND GENDER IDENTIFICATION

The issue of "Why am I lesbian, gay, bisexual, or transgendered?" is quite likely to arise in treatment. Some individuals who have been sexually abused in childhood frame their sexual orientation or gender identification in a reductionist and self-denigrating way, as the outcome of their abuse experiences. Unfortunately, they are likely to be encouraged in this way of thinking by relatives, friends, clergy, and even some mental health professionals, who see their sexual orientation and/or gender identification as one more terrible problem in their blighted lives.

Therapists of LGBT people have the responsibility to develop an educated perspective on the origins of sexual orientation and gender identification, independent of the perspective the client brings to treatment. Though much, of course, can be learned from listening to one's client, therapists whose only source of knowledge about LGBT people is what their clients tell them are unlikely to be able to create an empowering context in which these clients can struggle with their difficulties. A client might declare with utter conviction and sincerity that he knows he will no longer experience the sexual feelings for other men that he has felt since early adolescence when he has dealt with his abuse experience in therapy. A therapist who does not know enough to caution the client that this is unlikely to be the case and who in any way reinforces what is, in the vast majority of cases, wishful thinking, is colluding with the client in his internalized homophobia and is implicitly making promises about the therapy process that cannot be kept. Such a treatment will eventually lead to further self-hatred and despair.

There are still some mental health professionals who are working with lesbian, gay, bisexual, and transgendered clients who interpret their clients' attraction to people of the same sex or inability to conform to gender-identity norms as pathological (Falco, 1991; Fox, 1995; Silverstein, 1991). Some even counsel that to find happiness their clients must cure their deviant patterns of arousal or re-shape their sense of gender identity. Even a relatively recently published book about personality disorders (Akhtar, 1992) proffers outdated psychoanalytic dogma about gender and sexuality, as if these were scientific observations rather than the expression of a set of cultural attitudes and values:

> A cohesive gender identity is concordant with one's biological sex and shows harmony between core gender identity, gender role, and sexual partner orientation. This translates into heterosexual object choice and an overall gender-appropriate demeanor including attire, gestures, roles, social priorities, sexual behaviors, and interpersonal relationships. (pp. 35-36)

Even when professionals do not go so far as to advocate a change in gender identity, sexual desire, or object choice, they may see any fantasies, desires, and practices with which they are not personally familiar as deviant, thus colluding in disciplining clients to conform to narrow social standards. A wide array of activities–including cross-dressing, polyamory, and enactments of sexual fantasies (for example, domination/submission)–are frequently discounted by mental health professionals as *de facto* pathological. Therapists should make every effort to learn about differences in sexual practices or gender expression before assuming that all such differences are psychological problems to be altered through therapeutic intervention.

Therapists are frequently taught that sexual orientation is a stable and fundamental aspect of an individual's identity, and there are some interesting studies in three disciplines–neuroanatomy, endocrinology, and genetics–that examine the ways in which biology may play a part in the development of sexual orientation in some individuals (LeVay, 1991; Hamer, Hu, Magneson, Hu, & Pattatucci, 1995; Money, 1987; Swaab, Gooran, & Hofman, 1992; Kirk, Baily, Dunn, & Martin, 2000; Dawood, Pillard, Horvath, Revelle, & Bailey, 2000; Bailey, Dunne, & Martin, 2000; Pillard & Bailey, 1998; Herron & Herron, 1996). Every new study tends to be hailed as if the results offer a simple answer to a simple question, but so far there are no data that point to genes, life experience, or brain morphology as the sole and simple source for the many variations in the ways in which sexual desire, longing for affiliation, and gender identity manifest themselves in different people. Clients have a right to hold whatever opinion suits them about the subject. It is, however, incumbent upon mental health professionals to inform ourselves, so that we do not unintentionally implant or reinforce damaging views that are not empirically supported.

GENDER AND SEXUALITY EXPRESSED THROUGH DISSOCIATIVE STATES

Individuals who have been the victims of severe and chronic childhood abuse, including child sexual abuse, frequently develop dissociative defenses to enable them to manage what they cannot escape or understand. As adults, severely dissociative individuals often express their experiences and understanding of their sexuality and gender identity rigidly in concrete and demarcated states of consciousness that they may experience as male, female, gay, straight, and bisexual.

Exploring a patient's self-identifications in terms of both gender and sexual orientation can offer both patient and therapist a wider and deeper understanding of some of the patient's core therapeutic issues.

Unpacking individuals' beliefs as they are manifest in personality states can be illuminative of the evolution of their sexuality and gender identity in many ways. In 1989, I distributed questionnaires about dissociative states and sexual expression to a small number of individuals diagnosed at that time as suffering from multiple personality disorder (Rivera, 1996). The responses illustrated the richness and diversity of the pathways that these people traveled in developing their understanding of themselves as gendered and sexual. Respondents were asked to explore their views, attitudes, and behavior regarding sexuality as expressed in altered states of consciousness. As the questionnaire was long and detailed, only individuals who experienced gender and sexuality as significant issues for them would have been likely to have filled it out. Given that I did not select by sexual orientation, it is interesting that all of the questionnaires that were returned were from individuals who either identified as lesbian (N = 10) or gay male (N = 2), or who identified as bisexual (N = 8, all female).

I did not conclude that more severely dissociative abuse survivors were gay than straight from this small and not particularly randomly selected group of individuals seen in my practice, the practices of a few colleagues, or who attended a local self-help group or attended a forum "For Multiples Only" at a dissociation conference held in Toronto. In fact, research indicates that the same percentage of women who self-identify as lesbians have a history of childhood sexual abuse–38% (Loulan, 1987)–as women in studies in which sexual orientation was not noted (Russell, 1986). I hypothesized that, for individuals struggling to understand their sexual desires, same-sex sexuality needed more explaining–and from severely dissociative people, more dividing up–to make it manageable than heterosexual sexuality.

The rich and detailed life stories that were written in response to the questionnaire illustrated the complexity of the construction of sexuality as it plays itself out in the lives of trauma survivors. The following were common configurations:

- Child personality states who wanted affection and were horrified when the affection turned sexual;
- Anhedonic states in which individuals experienced themselves as asexual and sometimes non-gendered as well;
- Hypersexual teenagers, sometimes promiscuous;
- Stereotypically heterosexual feminine personalities who voiced conventional desires for security, safety, and a vine-covered cottage and saw sex as a means to those ends;

- Male-identified personalities in women's bodies who were actively sexual with other women and framed the behavior as heterosexual;
- Female-identified personalities in men's bodies who were passively sexual with other men and framed the behavior as heterosexual;
- Sexually aggressive personalities in both lesbians and gay men, usually experienced as male by both women and men;
- Personalities who knew they were lesbian or gay and were comfortable with that awareness;
- Personalities who thought it was silly to choose the people to whom you wanted to relate intimately by whether they were men or women, rather than by what they were like in so many other ways.

There were scores of permutations and combinations of personality states with different self-understandings about their gender and sexual identity in the twenty questionnaires that were fully filled out. The respondents (N = 5) who had had a lot of therapy and appeared to have resolved a great many of the most dysfunctional aspects of their dissociative coping mechanisms described the evolution of their understandings about their sexuality. Some personalities who had endorsed stereotypical (and often viciously intolerant) perspectives about same-sex sexual expression as an unnatural (and usually ungodly) abomination became more accepting of the desires and the practices of the others. Eventually, in the less rigidly divided person, earlier self-loathing about same-sex relationships was replaced with general acceptance and only the occasional deprecatory self-judgment. Child personalities were gradually subsumed into the general category of childlikeness or vulnerability, and those aspects of the individual, as described by some individuals, disappeared during sexual activity or, as described by others, became a playful aspect of sexual expression.

By termination, clients who complete a thorough and successful psychotherapy process usually resolve much of their confusion and dividedness about gender and sexuality. The assertiveness that initially could only be expressed when the individual experienced herself as a man becomes increasingly integrated with the sensitivity and vulnerability that she has always associated with femininity and has expressed in personality states she understands to be female. Gradually, (at least for those who are not transgendered) gender issues become less central and only occasionally emerge from the background. Most integrated individuals come to experience some degree of comfort with their biological sex, their gender identity, and their sexual orientation.

TRANSGENDER: CHALLENGING ASSUMPTIONS ABOUT GENDER

Our diagnostic system assumes that those who are not willing or not able to conform to our gender-identity norms have a mental disorder. However, we have not yet validated this assumption, and, in fact, the research that has been conducted thus far (Cole et al., 1997; Haraldsen & Dahl, 2000) contradicts it. At present, such framing of the transgendered person's experience of him/herself as a psychiatric disorder ("gender identity disorder") is ideological, rather than being based on any empirical data. It has its roots in genderism, the belief that there are only two genders that are natural and that everyone's gender identity should match his or her biological sex. Thus far, there is no evidence that transsexuality is psychopathological; the category "gender identity disorder" simply refers to a difference in the experience of gender identity from the norm. Until there is empirical validation for the link between a transgendered identity and psychopathology, the diagnostic category "gender identity disorder" is an expression of prejudice rather than a scientifically-based description of a mental illness. Surely, the medical community is capable of finding appropriate medical terminology to describe the need of some transsexuals for hormone therapy or sex re-assignment surgery that does not involve diagnosing patients who exhibit no psychiatric symptoms as mentally disordered! As with any other medical procedure, a psychiatric assessment can and should be ordered when there is evidence that mental illness may influence the patient's capacity to consent to treatment or to benefit from it.

Psychiatric medicine has a long history of creating linguistic categories that reify ethnocentric values that support exclusions and oppression. In the antebellum southern United States, for example, Samuel Cartwright, a highly respected and widely published medical doctor, invented the disorder, "drapetomania," defined as "the morbid compulsion to be free." This category was applied to slaves who tried to escape from captivity. In Cartwright's popular article (1851/1967), "Diseases and Peculiarities of the Negro Race," such slaves were not only seen as disobeying the law that bound them as property to their owners but as mentally ill for experiencing a desire that was socially unacceptable at the time. Dr. Cartwright offers this advice to slave owners, "With the advantages of proper medical advice, strictly followed, this troublesome practice that many Negroes have of running away can be almost entirely prevented" (http://www.pbs.org/wgbh/aia/part4/4h3106.html).

To date, no empirical evidence suggests a need to treat gender identity dysphoria as a mental disorder. Could it be that, like the creation of the category "drapetomania," the need to define difference in gender identity and presentation as a mental disorder may be nothing more than a reflection of social prejudices? It is our responsibility as social scientists to learn from the history of our profession and avoid creating and reinforcing diagnostic categories that reify bias and further marginalize those who challenge social norms to which most of us conform without much thought or effort.

Individuals' gender identity is usually established at an early age, and most transgendered individuals are the targets of pervasive discrimination throughout childhood. The markers of their biological sex are usually a source of great distress to them. They are frequently pressured or even forced into dress and activities that are profoundly ego-dystonic, as a routine part of sex-role socialization. Forcing a child who experiences his gender to be male to wear a dress or a child who thinks of herself as a girl to participate in an all-boy hockey league exacerbates their pervasive sense of shame and highlights their need to hide from others who they are. As they grow older, most find ways to accommodate their cross-gender identity to increase their own comfort level without risking the loss of their social status and all that goes with it, including family acceptance, jobs, intimate partnerships, and children. Many of these individuals struggle daily to find just the line of gender expression in dress and stance so that they can be somewhat comfortable with how they present themselves to the world without risking constant social censure.

One transgendered man described in a group therapy session an encounter with a young child and her mother on the street. "Hi, man," the little girl spoke to him cheerfully. He smiled and was about to greet her in response, feeling happy to meet such an outgoing, confident child, when the mother grabbed her daughter's hand and pulled her away, saying, "That's not a man, and don't talk to her." He continued walking on home, trying to cover his shame and sadness with anger. "It always happens," he muttered to the group, "It always happens."

Some transgendered individuals eventually choose to be open about their gender identity. This can be a great relief, just as lesbians, gays, and bisexuals experience a sense of liberation when they decide they will no longer hide their sexual orientation. However, coming out as a transgendered person can be even more fraught with social peril than coming out as gay, lesbian, or bisexual. Many people feel perfectly free to contest the gender identity of a transgendered individual. "You look just like a woman; I never would have known you are not one." "You may not come into this shelter; it is only for real women, women who were born women." The refusal to use the name or the pronouns that the person prefers is one of the ways in which this discomfort can be expressed by family, friends, and sometimes therapists as well.

Transgendered men and women often experience their childhood abuse as being related to their inability to fit into gender stereotypes. One transgendered man, brought up as a girl with three sisters, was certain that his father had anal sex with him for ten years because he was a boy, but a boy with female body parts. His experience of himself as a boy pre-dated the abuse, but the abuse reinforced his sense of shame about his body and his conviction that this was the type of treatment he could expect, and perhaps deserved, for having a body that did not match who he was.

The individual solutions offered to people suffering from a profound disruption between their bodies and their sense of themselves as gendered tend to perpetuate the denial that is at the heart of the transgendered person's dysphoria. Post-operative transsexuals are often advised to invent a new childhood for themselves and to destroy all evidence of their previous sex. As Kate Bornstein (1994) notes, "Transexuality is the only condition for which the therapy is to lie" (p. 62). Proposed societal solutions, such as "gender doesn't matter," implicitly or explicitly criticize transgendered people as gender conformists and facilely deny the felt reality of their personal torment. Transcending the constraints of gender (or playing at doing so when it suits us) is a luxury of those who have a comfortable sense of gender identity that conforms to social norms and very little recognition of the many ways in which we ourselves participate in the maintenance of a strict sex/gender social system (MacDonald, 1998).

Therapists of transgendered women and men must be open to the wide range of healthy gender and sexual expression if we are to help our clients deal with their experience, past and present, of living in a society that is not accepting of their expression of gender identity. Without extending our own knowledge base, challenging our own preconceptions, and widening our empathic capacity, we are in danger of becoming one more source of oppression in our transgendered clients' lives by framing as problematic and a target for therapeutic change what may be utterly core to their sense of self.

Gender issues are often difficult for many severely dissociative trauma survivors, those who are transgendered and the majority who are not. Most individuals suffering from Dissociative Identity Disorder have personality states in which they experience themselves as cross-gendered (Putman et al., 1986; Ross et al., 1989), and daily conflicts about what clothes to wear to present oneself as appropriately masculine or feminine are very common. By termination, clients frequently resolve their confusion and dividedness about their gender, and they come to experience some degree of congruence between their biological sex and their gender identity. The assertiveness that initially can only be expressed when the individual experiences herself as a man becomes increasingly integrated with the sensitivity and vulnerability that she has always associated with femininity and has expressed in personality states she understands to be female. Gradually, gender issues become less central and only occasionally emerge from the background.

Transgendered individuals who suffer from Dissociative Identity Disorder may well also experience gradually less confusion and dividedness regarding gender identity as they make some gains in therapy, but they experience increasing certainty that their gender is not congruent with their biological sex. Some may choose to undergo sex-reassignment surgery, but for many this is not desirable or even possible. Some gender identity clinics exclude individuals with a history of mental illness. Others do not consider a psychiatric disorder a contraindication for sex re-assignment surgery or hormone treatment, as long as the clients' perspectives regarding gender identity do not fluctuate with the psychiatric disorder and they are reasonably stable emotionally (Benjamin, 2001; Brown & Rounsely, 1996).

There has been no published research on the topic of treatment outcomes for DID clients who are transgendered, although there are two published case studies on individuals who were diagnosed with severe dissociative disorders after they had undergone sex-reassignment surgery (Saks, 1998; Schwartz, 1988). I have worked with a small number of dissociative individuals who have consolidated cross-gendered identities (sometimes with periodic hormone therapy and always without surgery). They each found a way to come to terms with themselves as transgendered and to make reasoned choices they could live with relatively peacefully.

One transgendered man officially changed his name from one that identified him as a female, transformed his appearance through a combination of a hormone regimen and replacing all clothes that were even slightly feminine, and gradually lived life openly as a man. As there were no employment issues for him to consider, and his children were tolerant of his transformation, he was able to be open about his experience of himself as a man. However, rather than denying his history (as is often recommended in gender identity clinics as part of the process of cross-gender transformation), he acknowledges that the parts of him whom he had experienced as female are valuable aspects of who he is, and he works at incorporating his feminine qualities into his sense of himself as a man who is both assertive and tender.

A transgendered woman, who works in a traditionally male job where stereotypically masculine qualities are privileged and any open gender ambiguity would be not only scorned but dangerous, chooses to live a bifurcated life. At work, she is as tough as the job requires. At home, she lives her life as a woman. She seems no more conflicted about her way of life than many individuals who have to be less authentic at work than they would like to have a successful career, and though she gets considerable satisfaction from her challenging job, she also looks forward to retirement and a move to a different city where she will be free to live more fully as a woman.

In both of these cases, the basic consolidation of a cross-gendered identity occurred long before all the issues related to their trauma histories and dissociative adaptations had been unearthed and resolved in the therapeutic process. The relief and well-being that came from acknowledging and living out their transgendered identity appeared to give these individuals the confidence eventually to explore extremely difficult issues more fully and deeply.

DID AND GENDER IDENTITY DISORDER–DIFFERENTIAL DIAGNOSIS

When assessing gender dysphoric individuals presenting for hormone treatment or sex re-assignment surgery, who have a history of childhood trauma and report or exhibit signs of psychopathology, it is extremely important that physicians and mental health professionals consider a dissociative disorder, and particularly Dissociative Identity Disorder (DID), in their differential diagnosis (Brown & Rounsley, 1996; Devor, 1994; Saks, 1998; Schwartz, 1988). Though a history of trauma and a dissociative disorder do not preclude genuine transexuality, any radical and irreversible treatment should only be undertaken with the full awareness of its life-altering effects. Informed consent cannot be provided by a client who is unaware of his or her beliefs, experiences, and behaviors in dissociated states of consciousness, or who is unwilling to explore them. Saks (1998) recounts the case history of a biological female who had developed a dissociative disorder in response to severe childhood abuse. In adulthood, two male alter personalities dominated for eleven years, during which the individual cross-dressed, lived as a man most of the time, and passed all the psychological tests to qualify for sex re-assignment surgery, consciously hiding from the clinic personnel information about her history of dissociative symptomatology. Three surgeries were performed, and ten years later the client had a mental breakdown during which Dissociative Identity Disorder was diagnosed. Alter personalities have emerged in subsequent treatment who understand themselves as girls and women, presumably creating significant internal conflict about the surgically-altered body. Schwartz (1988) reports the case of a post-operative female transexual who was diagnosed with multiple personality disorder years after sex reassignment surgery. Although in this case the male alter personalities concurred with the decision to be female, Schwartz cautions that it is crucial to uncover and treat dissociative disorders before recommending surgery.

CONCLUSION

This article touches on only a few of the issues that mental health professionals treating lesbians, gay, bisexual, and transgendered clients with trauma histories may face over the course of psychotherapy. There is very little published on the treatment of lesbian, gay, bisexual, and transgendered clients with dissociative disorders. This is an important area for the creation of constructive theory, the publishing of clinical experience, and the development of research studies that will enable the mental health profession in general, and the trauma and dissociation field in particular, to practice more sensitively and effectively with our lesbian, gay, bisexual, and transgendered clients.

REFERENCES

Akhtar, S. (1992). *Broken structures: Severe personality disorders and their treatment.* Northvale, NJ: Jason Aronson.

American Psychological Association. (1991). *Bias in psychotherapy with lesbians and gay men: Final report of the task force on psychotherapy with lesbians and gay men.* Washington, DC: author.

American Psychological Association. *American Psychological Association guidelines for treating lesbian, gay and bisexual clients*. www.apa.org.

Bailey, J.M., Dunne, M.P., & Martin, N.G. (2000). Genetic and environmental influences on sexual orientation and its correlates in an Australian twin sample. *Journal of Personal and Social Psychology, 78*, 524-536.

Bell, A. & Weinberg, M. (1978). *Homosexualities: A study of diversity among men and women*. New York: Simon and Schuster.

Benjamin, H. (1966). *The transsexual phenomenon*. New York: Julian Press.

Benjamin, H. (2001). *The Harry Benjamin International Gender Dysphoria Association's standards of care for gender identity disorder, Sixth version*. www.hbigda.org/socv6.html.

Bergler, E. (1956). *Homosexualities: Disease or new way of life?* New York: Collier Books.

Bieschke, K.J., McClanahan, M., Tozer, E., Grzegorek, J.L, & Park, J. (2000). Programmatic research on the treatment of lesbian, gay, and bisexual clients: The past, the present, and the course of the future. In R.M. Perez, K.A. DeBord, & K.J. Bieschke, (Eds). *Handbook of counselling and psychotherapy with lesbian, gay, and bisexual clients* (pp. 309-336). Washington, DC: American Psychological Association.

Blumstein, P., & Schwartz, P. (1989). Bisexuality: Some social psychological issues. *Journal of Social Issues, 33*(2), 30-45.

Bornstein, K. (1994). *Gender outlaw: On men, women, and the rest of us*. New York: Routledge.

Bieschke, K.J., & Matthews, C. (1996). Career counselor attitudes and behaviors toward gay, lesbian, and bisexual clients. *Journal of Vocational Behavior, 48*, 243-255.

Brown, L.S. (1995). Lesbian identities: Concepts and issues. In A.R. D'Augelli, & CJ. Patterson (Eds.), *Lesbian, gay, and bisexual identities over the lifespan: Psychological perspectives over the lifespan* (pp. 3-23). New York: Oxford University Press.

Brown, L.S. (1989). New voices, new visions: Toward a lesbian/gay paradigm for psychology. *Psychology of Women Quarterly, 13*, 445-458.

Brown, M., & Rounsley, C. (1996). *Understanding transexualism: For families, friends, co-workers, and helping professionals*. San Francisco: Jossey-Bass Publishers.

Buhrke, R., & Douce, L. (1991). Training issues for counseling psychologists in working with lesbian women and gay men. *The Counseling Psychologist, 19*, 216-234.

Caprio, F. (1954). *Female homosexuality: A psychodynamic study of lesbianism*. New York: Citadel Press.

Cartwright, S. (1851/1967). Diseases and peculiarities of the Negro race. *DeBow's Review, Southern and Western States, 11*. New York: AMS Press. http://www.pbs.org/wgbh/aia/part4/4h3106.html (1 Feb. 2002).

Clark, W., & Serovich, J. (1997). Twenty years and still in the dark? Content analysis of articles pertaining to gay, lesbian, and bisexual issues in marriage and family therapy journals. *Journal of Marital and Family Therapy, 23*, 239-253.

Cole, C., O'Boyle, M., Emery, L., & Meyer, W. (1997). Comorbidity of gender dysphoria and other major psychiatric diagnoses. *Archives of Sexual Behavior, 26*(1), 13-26.

Cope, A. & Darke, J. (1999). *Trans accessibility project: Making women's shelters accessible to transgendered women*. Toronto, Canada: Violence and Intervention and Education Workgroup, Ontario Ministry of Education and Training.

D`Augelli, A.R., & Patterson, C.J. (1995). *Lesbian, gay and bisexual identities over the lifespan: Psychological perspectives*. New York: Oxford University Press.

Dawood, K., Pillard, R.C., Horvath, C., Revelle, W., & Bailey, J.M. (2000). Familial aspects of male homosexuality. *Archives of Sexual Behavior, 29*(2), 155-163.

DeBord, K.A., & Perez, R.M. (2000). Group counseling theory and practice with lesbian, gay, and bisexual clients. In R. M. Perez, K.A. DeBord, & K.J. Bieschke (Eds.), *Handbook of counselling and psychotherapy with lesbian, gay, and bisexual clients* (pp. 183-206). Washington, DC: American Psychological Association.

Devor, H. (1994). Transsexualism, dissociation, and child abuse: An initial discussion based on non-clinical data. *Journal of Psychology and Human Sexuality, 6*(3), 49-72.

Devor, H. (1997). *Female to male transexuals in society*. Bloomington, IN: Indiana University Press.

Downey, J., & Friedman, R. (1995). Internalized homophobia in lesbian relationships. *Journal of the American Academy of Psychoanalysis, 23*, 435-447.

Ellis, A. (1965). *Homosexuality: Its causes and cure*. New York: Lyle Stuart.

Falco, K. (1991). *Psychotherapy with lesbian clients: Theory into practice*. New York: Brunner/Mazel.

Feinberg, L. (1993). *Stone Butch Blues*. Ithaca, NY: Firebrand Books.

Feinberg, L. (1996). *Transgender warriors: Making history from Joan of Arc to RuPaul*. Boston: Beacon Press.

Fox, R. (1995). Bisexuality identities. In A. D'Augelli, & C. Patterson (Eds.), *Lesbian, gay and bisexual identities over the lifespan* (pp. 48-86). New York: Oxford University Press.

Group for the Advancement of Psychiatry (2000). *Homosexuality and the Mental Health Professions*. Hillsdale, NJ: The Analytic Press.

Garnets, L., & Kimmel, D. (1991). Lesbian and gay male dimensions in the psychological study of human diversity. In. J.D. Goodchilds (Ed.), *Psychological perspectives on human diversity in America* (pp. 137-189). Washington, DC: American Psychological Association.

Garnets, L., & Kimmel, D. (Eds.). (1993). *Psychological perspective on lesbian and gay male experiences*. New York: Columbia University Press.

Gelso, C., Fassinger, R., Gomez, M., & Latts, M. (1995). Countertransference reactions to lesbian clients: The role of homophobia, counselor gender, and countertransference management. *Journal of Counseling Psychology, 42*, 356-364.

Gonsiorek, J.C., & Rudolph, J.R. (1991) Homosexual identity: Coming out and other developmental events. In J.C. Gonsiorek, & J.W. Weinrich, (Eds.). *Homosexuality: Research implications for public policy* (pp. 161-176). Newbury Park, CA: Sage Publications.

Gottman, J. (1989). Children of gay and lesbian parents. *Marriage and Family Review, 14*, 177-196.

Green, C.D., & Bozett, F.W. (1991). Lesbian mothers and gay fathers. In J. Gonsiorek, & J. Weinrich (Eds.), *Homosexuality: Research implications for public policy* (pp. 197-214). Newbury Park, CA: Sage Publications.

Green, R. (1996). Why ask, why tell? Teaching and learning about lesbians and gays in family therapy. *Family Process, 35*, 389-400.

Griggs, C. (1998). *S/he: Changing sex and changing clothes*. New York: Berg.

Hamer, D., Hu, S., Magneson, V., Hu, V., & Pattatucci, A. (1995). A Linkage between DNA markers on the X chromosome and male sexual orientation. *Science, 261*, 321-327.

Hancock, K.A. (1995). Psychotherapy with lesbians and gay men. In A. D'Augelli, & C. Patterson, (Eds.). *Lesbian, gay, and bisexual identities over the lifespan* (pp. 323-336). New York: Oxford University Press.

Haraldsen, I., & Dahl, A. (2000). Symptom profiles of gender dysphoric patients of transsexual type compared to patients with personality disorders and healthy adults. *Acta Psychiatra Scandinavia, 102*(4), 276-281.

Hayes, J.A., & Gelso, C.J. (1993). Male counselors' discomfort with gay and HIV-infected clients. *Journal of Counseling Psychology, 40*, 86-93.

Herron, W.G., & Herron, M.J. (1996). The complexity of sexuality. *Psychological Reports, 78*(1), 129-130.

Holahan, W., & Gibson, S.A. (1994). Heterosexual therapists leading lesbian and gay therapy groups. Therapeutic and political realities. *Journal of Counseling & Development, 72*, 591-594.

Hooker, E. (1957). The adjustment of the male homosexual. *Journal of Projective Techniques, 21*, 18-31.

Hopkins, J.H. (1969). The lesbian personality. *British Journal of Psychiatry, 115*, 1433-1436.

Israel, G., & Tarver, D. (1997). *Transgender Care*. Philadelphia: Temple University Press.

Kinsey, A.C., Pomeroy, W.B., & Martin, C.E. (1948). *Sexual behavior in the human male*. Philadelphia: W.B. Saunders.

Kinsey, A.C., Pomeroy, W.B., Martin, C.E., & Gebhard, P. (1953). *Sexual behavior in the human female*. Philadelphia: W.B. Saunders.

Kirk, K.M., Bailey, J.M., Dunne, M.P., & Martin, N.G. (2000). Measurement models for sexual orientation in a community twin sample. *Behavioral Genetics, 30*, 345-356.

Klein, F., Sepekoff, B., & Wolf, T.J. (1985). Sexual orientation: A multi-variable dynamic process. *Journal of Homosexuality, 11*(1/2), 35-49.

LeVay, S. (1991). A difference in hypothalamic structure between heterosexual and homosexual men. *Science, 253*, 1034-1037.

Lewis, K. (1980). Children of lesbians: their point of view. *Social Work, May*, 198-203.

Loulan, J. (1987). *Lesbian passion: Loving ourselves and each other*. Duluth, MN: Spinsters INK.

MacDonald, E. (1998). Critical Identities: Rethinking feminism through transgender politics. *Atlantis, 23*(1), 190-197.

McHenry, S.S., & Johnson, J.W. (1993). Homophobia in the therapist and gay or lesbian client: Conscious and unconscious collusions in self-hate. *Psychotherapy, 30*, 141-151.

Money, J. (1987). Sin, sickness, or status? Homosexual gender identity and psychoneuroendocrinology. *American Psychologist*, *42*, 384-99.

Morrow, S.L., Gore, P.A., & Campbell, B.W. (1996). The application of a sociocognitive framework to the career development of lesbians and gay men. *Journal of Vocational Behavior*, *48*, 136-148.

Moses, A.E., & Hawkins, R.O. (1982). *Counseling lesbian women and gay men.* Columbus, OH: Mosby.

Namaste, K. (1998). The everyday bisexual as problematic: Research methods beyond monosexism. In J.L. Ristock, & C.G. Taylor, (Eds.) *Inside the academy and out: Lesbian/gay/queer studies and social action.* Toronto: University of Toronto Press.

Ossama, S.M. (2000). Relationship and couples counselling. In R.M. Perez, K.A. DeBord, & K.J. Bieschke (Eds.), *Handbook of counselling and psychotherapy with lesbian, gay, and bisexual clients* (pp. 275-302). Washington, DC: American Psychological Association.

Perez, R.M., DeBord, K.A., & Bieschke, K.J. (Eds.) (2000). *Handbook of counselling and psychotherapy with lesbian, gay and bisexual clients.* Washington, DC: American Psychological Association.

Phillips, J.C. (2000). Training issues and considerations. In R.M. Perez, K.A. DeBord, & K.J. Bieschke (Eds.), *Handbook of counselling and psychotherapy with lesbian, gay, and bisexual clients* (pp. 337-358). Washington, DC: American Psychological Association.

Pillard, R.C., & Bailey, J.M. (1998). Human sexual orientation has a heritable component. *Human Biology*, *70*, 347- 365.

Putman, F.W., Guroff, J.J. Silberman, E.K., Barban., L., & Post, R.M. (1986). The clinical phenomenology of multiple personality disorder: Review of 100 recent cases. *Journal of Clinical Psychiatry*, *47*, 172-175.

Rivera, M. (1996). Treatment of lesbian and gay survivors of abuse. In M. Rivera, *More alike than different: Treating severely dissociative trauma survivors* (pp. 190-208). Toronto: University of Toronto Press.

Rivera, M., & Wachob, S. (in press). Treatment of gay, lesbian, bisexual, and transgender survivors of child sexual abuse. In L.E.A. Walker, S.W. Gold, & B.A. Lucenko (Eds.), *Handbook on sexual abuse of children: Assessment, treatment & legal issues.* New York: Springer.

Ross, C.A., Norton, G.R., & Wozney, K. (1989). Multiple personality disorder: An analysis of 236 cases. *Canadian Journal of Psychiatry*, *34*, 413-418.

Roth, S. (1985). Psychotherapy with lesbian couples: Individual issues, female socialization, and the social context. In. M. McGoldrick, C. Anderson, & F. Walsh (Eds.), *Women in families: A framework for family therapy* (pp. 286-307). New York: Norton.

Rubin, G. (1984). Thinking sex: Notes for a radical theory of the politics of sexuality. In C. Vance (Ed.), *Pleasure and danger: Exploring female sexuality* (pp. 300-309). Boston: Routledge and Kegan Paul.

Russell, D.E.H. (1986). *The secret trauma. Incest in the lives of girls and women.* New York: Basic Books.

Saks, B.M. (1998). Transgenderism and dissociative identity disorder: A case study. *The International Journal of Transgenderism*, *2*(2), http://www.symposion.com/ijt/ijtc0404.htm.

Schwartz, P.G. (1988). A case of concurrent multiple personality disorder and transsexualism. *Dissociation*, *1*(2), 48-51.

Silverstein, C. (1991). Psychological and medical treatments of homosexuality. In J.C. Gonsiorek, & J.D. Weinrach (Eds.), *Homosexuality: Research implications for public policy* (pp. 101-114). Newbury Park, CA: Sage.

Socarides, C. (1968). *The overt homosexual*. New York: Grune & Stratton.

Swaab, D.F., Gooran, L.J., & Hofman, M.A. (1992). Gender and sexual orientation in relation to hypothalamic structures. *Hormone Research*, *38*, 51-61.

Thompson, N.L., McCandless, B.R., & Strickland, B.R. (1971). Personal adjustment of male and female homosexuals and heterosexuals. *Journal of Abnormal Psychology*, *78*, 237-240.

Troiden, R.R. (1989). The formation of homosexual identities. *Journal of Homosexuality*, *17*, 43-73.

Weinberg, M., Williams, C., & Pryor, D. (1994). *Dual attraction: Understanding Bisexuality*. New York: Oxford University Press.

Dissociation and Sexual Addiction/Compulsivity: A Contextual Approach to Conceptualization and Treatment

Steven N. Gold, PhD
Robert E. Seifer, MS

SUMMARY. The possible relationship of dissociation to sexual addiction/compulsivity (SAC) among childhood sexual abuse (CSA) survivors is explored. In applying a treatment procedure based on functional behavioral analysis to CSA survivors exhibiting SAC it was frequently observed that SAC patterns of behavior were not sexually gratifying, but that clients had been previously unaware of this. These clients often had poor recall of even recent instances of SAC and described a subjective sense of being in a daze, truncated awareness, and absence of a sense of agency during SAC episodes. Repeated detailed description of recent incidents of SAC in session helped clients become less dissociative when subsequently participating in SAC behaviors and gradually reduced the appeal of engaging in them. On the basis of these observations it is ar-

Steven N. Gold and Robert E. Seifer are affiliated with the Trauma Resolution and Integration Program, Nova Southeastern University, Ft. Lauderdale, FL.

Address correspondence to: Steven N. Gold, PhD, Center for Psychological Studies, Nova Southeastern University, 3301 College Avenue, Fort Lauderdale, FL 33314 (E-mail: gold@nova.edu).

The authors wish to express their appreciation to Christine Courtois, PhD for her extremely helpful suggestions for improving this paper.

[Haworth co-indexing entry note]: "Dissociation and Sexual Addiction/Compulsivity: A Contextual Approach to Conceptualization and Treatment." Gold, Steven N., and Robert E. Seifer. Co-published simultaneously in *Journal of Trauma & Dissociation* (The Haworth Medical Press, an imprint of The Haworth Press, Inc.) Vol. 3, No. 4, 2002, pp. 59-82; and: *Trauma and Sexuality: The Effects of Childhood Sexual, Physical, and Emotional Abuse on Sexuality Identity and Behavior* (ed: James A. Chu, and Elizabeth S. Bowman) The Haworth Medical Press, an imprint of The Haworth Press, Inc., 2002, pp. 59-82. Single or multiple copies of this article are available for a fee from The Haworth Document Delivery Service [1-800-HAWORTH, 9:00 a.m. - 5:00 p.m. (EST). E-mail address: getinfo@haworthpressinc.com].

gued that recognition of the dissociative quality of SAC behavior in CSA survivors is essential to adequately understanding it, and that targeting the dissociative elements of SAC in treatment is crucial to disrupting it. It is also proposed that in this clinical population SAC can reflect the dissociative disconnectedness represented by re-enactment of CSA experiences, failure to integrate emotional intimacy with sexuality due to insecure or disorganized attachment, association of sexual activity with soothing and validation rather than sexual arousal, or a combination of these factors.

KEYWORDS. Dissociation, childhood sexual abuse. sexual addiction, psychotherapy, functional behavioral analysis

It is unquestionably the case that childhood sexual abuse (CSA) is a topic around which a substantial body of professional literature has developed since the 1980s. Sexual addiction and compulsivity (SAC) has similarly been a subject about which progressively more has been written in recent years. However, although several authors have noted a relationship between CSA and SAC (e.g., Carnes & Delmonico, 1996; Courtois, 1988; Hunter & Struve, 1998; Whitfield, 1998), relatively little detailed exploration of this association has occurred to date. Similarly, while there is some mention in the literature of dissociative features in SAC (e.g., Schwartz & Southern, 2000; Whitfield, 1998), minimal conceptual elaboration on the mechanisms underlying this connection has been conducted. Our aim here is to explore the possible nature of the relationship between CSA and SAC, to consider in particular how dissociation may represent a point of connection between CSA and SAC, and to discuss the implications of this conceptual framework for treatment.

Dissociation and childhood sexual abuse (CSA) are phenomena that have come to be widely thought of as closely related to each other. Both phenomena were the object of considerable interest at the close of the 19th century, were largely neglected as areas of study during most of the 20th century, and were the subject of renewed attention in the closing decades of the 20th century. It is probably no coincidence that interest in these two topics has waxed and waned in tandem. CSA has come to be widely assumed to be a common etiological factor in the development of dissociative symptomatology; a fairly extensive body of empirical literature has developed consisting of evidence that has been for the most part supportive of this hypothesis (Anderson, Yasenik, & Ross, 1993; Chu & Dill, 1990; Kluft, 1990).

In addition to dissociation, there is a broad range of other symptom patterns and difficulties that have come to be considered possible long-term effects of CSA. These include: depression (Brown & Finkelhor, 1986); anxiety (Alexander, 1992, 1993; Mullen, Martin, Anderson, Romans, & Herbison, 1996), frequently manifested as posttraumatic stress disorder (PTSD; Rowan and Foy, 1993; Rodriguez, Ryan, Rowan, & Foy, 1996); somatic symptoms (McCauley et al., 1997); personality disorders (Herman, 1992; Herman, Perry, & van der Kolk, 1989; Perry, Herman, van der Kolk, & Holk, 1990); substance abuse (Bennett & Kemper, 1994; Brown & Finkelhor, 1986; Spak, Spak, & Allebeck, 1997; Wilsnack, Vogeltanz, Klassen, & Harris, 1997); eating disorders (de Groot & Rodin, 1999; Fallon & Wonderlich, 1997); self-mutilation (Lipschitz et al., 1999; Nijman et al., 1999); other addictive and compulsive patterns of behavior (Anderson & Coleman, 1991; Tedesco & Bola, 1997); and relationship difficulties (Courtois, 1988; Herman, 1992; Freyd, 1996). Clinically, one often finds several of these difficulties in combination with dissociative symptomatology in individuals seeking therapy who report a history of CSA (Anderson, Yasenik, & Ross, 1993; Chu & Dill, 1990; Kluft, 1990).

When one considers the relatively extensive spectrum of problems that have been associated with a background of CSA, it is striking how relatively little literature has addressed the impact of CSA on adult sexual functioning. One would think that one of the more obvious legacies of having been sexually molested in childhood might be the experience of difficulties in sexual adjustment later in life. However, this is an area of functioning that has received scant attention in both the empirical and clinical literature on CSA.

Literature on sexual difficulties among CSA survivors is limited, but it is by no means non-existent. Much of this literature is clinical in nature, a good deal of it is directed toward a popular rather than a professional audience, and the bulk of it focuses on women CSA survivors. The types of sexual difficulties frequently noted among women survivors are sexual dysfunction, anxiety about sex, flashbacks triggered by sexual activity, and dissociating during sexual encounters (Maltz, 1988, 1991; Maltz & Holman, 1987; Westerlund, 1983, 1992). The relatively few relevant empirical studies consistently indicate that the majority of CSA survivors report sexual and intimacy difficulties (Becker, Skinner,

Abel, & Cichon, 1986; Briere & Runtz, 1987; Courtois, 1988; Mackey et al., 1991). In a rare study comparing survivors of childhood sexual, physical and emotional abuse, problems with sexual functions were found to be significantly more prevalent among CSA survivors than among survivors of the other two forms of child abuse (Briere & Runtz, 1990).

A likely explanation for the limited exploration of this topic is that in light of the other pressing and potentially life-threatening problems frequently experienced by CSA survivors who enter therapy, sexual adjustment may appear to be a fairly low priority. Often clients with a CSA history present with a number of grave difficulties, such as intense and frequent distress, self-injury and other forms of self-destructive behavior, and severe dissociation that disrupts the capacity to maintain a sense of continuity and focus on the here and now. In comparison to problems of this magnitude, developing a gratifying sex life is likely to seem to be a relatively trivial concern, particularly if one assumes that the impact CSA most often has on sexual behavior is avoidance.

However, clinical observation may suggest otherwise. A substantial proportion of CSA survivor clients report patterns of sexual behavior that are repeatedly and persistently engaged in despite the fact that they carry severe negative consequences (Briere & Elliott, 1994; Courtois, 1988). Empirical research supports that participation in risky and impulsive sexual behavior is associated with a CSA history (e.g., Browning & Laumann, 1997; Cavaiola & Schiff, 1988; Dimock, 1988; Tsai, Feldman-Summers, & Edgar, 1979; Walser & Kern, 1996). We have observed this phenomenon at two demographically divergent settings: a community mental health center outpatient treatment program for CSA survivors that the first author directs–the Trauma Resolution & Integration Program (TRIP)–and in his independent practice. The outpatient program primarily serves a relatively indigent population, many whom are unemployed or on disability, while the clientele of the independent practice are residents of a relatively affluent suburban area. The patterns of sexual behavior described include activities such as the solicitation of prostitutes, anonymous sexual encounters with strangers picked up on the street or other public places, and spending hours at a time and large sums of money at strip clubs or at pornographic web sites. It is not the nature of these behaviors in and of itself that defines them as addictive or compulsive. What makes these activities problematic, and therefore identifies them as instances of SAC, is that they are repeatedly engaged in despite the high likelihood of encountering or in spite of already having actually sustained substantial penalties. These costs include the loss of a primary relationship when the behavior is discovered, expenditures of time and money in amounts so extensive that they interfere with employment and financial security, and contracting AIDS or other STDs through unprotected sex. The last of these risks highlights that SAC can be just as dire in its consequences as self-mutilation, which is more frequently recognized as being associated with a CSA history.

Both among CSA survivors and among those without a CSA history, men report engaging in SAC patterns of behavior much more often than do women. SAC appears, however, to be much more prevalent among men who are CSA survivors than among those who are not. We conservatively estimate that upwards of 70% of male CSA survivors in therapy acknowledge periods of engaging in SAC behaviors. (While a smaller proportion of women survivors complain of SAC, it was not a rarity for them either.) As has been noted elsewhere, the literature on the topics of CSA and dissociation is strongly focused on women, to the degree that often the very existence of men within these groups is largely ignored (Gill, 1999). Although men likely constitute the minority, they nevertheless comprise a significant proportion of CSA survivors (Briere, Evans, Runtz, & Wall, 1988; Dhaliwal, Gauzas, Antonowicz, & Ross, 1996; Finkelhor, 1990). The likelihood that SAC is more common among male than women survivors, and that male survivors have been a relatively neglected group, probably has contributed to the fact that SAC has not been widely addressed in the CSA literature.

Unfortunately, most of the existing knowledge base on SAC is derived almost exclusively from clinical observation. There is woefully little hard empirical research on SAC (Gold & Heffner, 1998). Despite the lack of substantial empirical support for the validity of the SAC construct, a sizeable network of institutions related to its treatment has been in existence for a number of years now. There are several specialized treatment programs for SAC throughout the U.S. An organization for professionals and treatment facilities specializing in SAC, the National Council on Sexual Addiction and Compulsivity (NCSAC, www.ncsac.org), was founded over a decade ago. NCSAC publishes its own journal, *Sexual Addiction & Compulsivity: The Journal of Treatment and Prevention* (London, UK: Taylor & Francis). However, the pieces in this journal consist almost exclusively of clinical and theoretical works, and very few empirical investigations of SAC have been published in other journals. Moreover, in large part due to the lack of empirical research to assess the validity of the diagnosis, SAC is not explicitly recognized in the DSM-IV (American Psychiatric Association, 1994).

To complicate the matter further, there is little overlap between the literature on SAC and the literature on CSA. Consequently, many individuals who specialize in each of these topics seem to have little familiarity with both of these subjects. There is therefore very little literature that explicitly addresses the possible relationship between these two areas. Although we have been developing a measure of SAC at TRIP in order to operationalize the construct and make it possible to do research on the relationship between CSA and SAC, this project is still in process and our findings are therefore only preliminary. For all these reasons, most of the material presented here is based on clinical observation and theory, and therefore should be considered preliminary and subject to empirical investigation.

The objectives of this article are to:

1. Introduce the reader to the construct of sexual addiction/compulsivity (SAC);
2. Describe a treatment protocol for SAC that was originally developed for dissociative CSA survivors;
3. Explore why SAC may be prevalent among CSA survivors; and
4. Delineate the ways in which SAC seems to be intimately related to dissociative processes.

WHAT IS SEXUAL ADDICTION/COMPULSIVITY (SAC)?

A major controversy in the literature on SAC revolved around the nature of this proposed disorder. Some authors argued that it was best considered an addiction (Carnes, 1983). Others insisted that it more closely approximated a compulsion (Allers, Benjack, White, & Rousey, 1993; Fischer, 1995; McCarthy 1994). A small minority alternately claimed that it was most accurately conceptualized as constituting an impulse control disorder (Levin & Troiden, 1988). The term "sexual addiction *and* compulsivity," which is incorporated both into the name of the professional organization NCSAC and its journal, reflects that a consensus was eventually reached that continued disputes about this issue were unlikely to be productive.

It would appear that a major reason for the controversy is that, in the absence of a DSM diagnosis specifically for SAC, this proposed syndrome can legitimately be construed as meeting the criteria comprising either an addictive disorder, an obsessive-compulsive disorder, or an impulse control disorder. SAC resembles an addictive disorder in that the same DSM-IV criteria that apply to substance dependence can be attributed to SAC (Goodman, 1992, 1993). These features of SAC include, for example, needing to engage in increasing amounts and extremes of sexual activity to obtain the desired effect (i.e., tolerance), repeated unsuccessful attempts to cut down on the activity, and sacrificing other aspects of living because of SAC activities. Similarly, SAC approximates obsessive-compulsive disorder in that it is often accompanied by obsessive preoccupation with sex, appears to serve the function of reducing anxiety, and can be (although certainly is not always, in our experience) ego-dystonic (Butts, 1992; Coleman, 1992; Earle and Crow 1990). SAC can also be classified as an impulse control disorder because like, for example, pathological gambling, it has many of the characteristics of a substance use disorder, but a behavior other than substance use is the source of difficulty (Barth and Kinder, 1987).

A crucial distinction in conceptualizing SAC is that unlike syndromes it may superficially appear to resemble that are associated with an earlier era, such as nymphomania and Don Juanism, the diagnosis is *not* primarily made on the basis of the frequency of sexual activity. Instead, the defining characteristic of SAC is that it consists of sexual behavior over which the individual does not experience a sense of control, and which consequently repeatedly creates social, occupational, or legal problems for her or him. There are a number of additional features that appear to be commonly associated with SAC as it is manifested among CSA survivors in particular, but which may not be typical of individuals with SAC who are not CSA survivors. Chief among these attributes is the presence of dissociative states while engaging in SAC behavior. The presence of this and other characteristics came to light in the course of employing a particular method of intervention originally developed for treating SAC among CSA survivors. Before discussing these features, therefore, it will be helpful to delineate this treatment approach.

SCAN-R: FUNCTIONAL BEHAVIORAL ANALYTIC TREATMENT OF SAC

The intervention method for SAC described here was developed as one component in a more comprehensive treatment approach for adult survivors of prolonged child abuse referred to as contextual therapy (Gold, 2000; in press). The specific procedure for reducing or eliminating SAC behavior within the course of contextual treatment is called

SCAN-R. SCAN-R is an acronym for the steps in the intervention: select, cue, analyze, note, and revise. It is, in effect, an application of the general principles of functional behavior analysis (Gold, 2000).

The SCAN-R procedure is introduced by explaining to the client that there will be no expectation or request to directly attempt to stop engaging in SAC behavior. Instead, it will be essential to commit to informing the therapist at the beginning of each session of any instances of SAC behavior since the previous meeting, and to be open to discussing them in detail. This is an agreement that clients are usually very willing to make, since the emphasis is not on giving up the behavior but on talking about it. Consequently, clients are unlikely to feel coerced by the therapist or to experience the therapeutic relationship as having adversarial undertones.

The first step in the SCAN-R procedure, to *select* an incident of SAC to discuss, is particularly essential to its success. It is imperative that discussion center on *a particular recent instance of SAC*, rather than on generalizations about the client's SAC behavior. One of the elements integral to the effectiveness of the SCAN-R procedure is that it directs the client's attention to aspects of the SAC behavior and of the circumstances associated with it of which she or he was not previously aware. Reliance on the client's impressionistic account of the SAC behavior is almost certain to fail to bring these elements to light. Only by closely examining particular instances of SAC is the client likely to identify facets of the SAC behavior pattern that did not previously capture her or his attention. Since the client has agreed to report any instances of SAC behavior, usually the episode discussed will be the most recent. This increases the likelihood that specific details of the incident will be accessible to recall.

Once the particular incident to be discussed has been identified, examination centers on clarifying the precursors of the behavior in an attempt to identify the *cues* that trigger engaging in SAC for the client. This is accomplished by asking the client questions such as:

> When did it first occur to you to do that (i.e., engage in the SAC behavior)? What was happening/what were you thinking about/what were you experiencing just before the idea to do that first occurred to you? What forethought or planning did you engage in before going ahead and acting on the decision to do that? What were you experiencing/feeling/thinking while planning it? How much time elapsed between when you first thought about engaging in that activity and when you made the decision to go ahead and do it? How

> much time elapsed between making the decision and acting on it? What was going on in between?

This type of inquiry serves several purposes. It helps to gradually bring into focus the types of events, thoughts, or feelings that trigger the sequence of behaviors that comprise the SAC pattern. This information, in turn, can eventually help the client to deduce the purpose of and motivations underlying SAC activity. Later in treatment, when the client may become more invested in relinquishing SAC behavior, recognition of the presence of these cues can serve as an early warning signal for initiating the use of relapse prevention strategies.

Once information regarding cues is obtained, questioning continues to help the client *analyze* the sequence of thoughts, feelings, behaviors and consequences that comprise the SAC episode once it is set in motion. This is accomplished by inquiring in intricate detail about the activities, circumstances, thoughts, and feelings associated with each phase of the incident as it unfolded. Typical queries in this phase of the procedure include:

> Once you decided to engage in the behavior, what was the very first thing you did to set things in motion? What were you thinking/experiencing/feeling as you did that? What were you thinking/experiencing/feeling right after you did that? What did you do/what happened next? What were you thinking/feeling as you did that/as that was happening? What were you thinking/feeling right after you did it/it happened?

This mode of inquiry should chronologically trace the entire course of the SAC episode up to and including its aftermath. This would mean, for instance, questioning such as:

> Once it was over, where did you go? What were you thinking and feeling during that time? What was the first thing you did when you got there? As you were doing that, what were you feeling? Thinking?

Throughout the phase of having the client *analyze* the incident, and immediately following inquiry about the particulars of the incident, the therapist facilitates having the client recognize or *note* nuances of the SAC pattern that were not apparent before. Once these elements are identified, the final phase of the procedure is to employ cognitive interventions to help the clients *revise* their previously held assumptions about the SAC activity on the basis of the newly noted features of the behavior. Clients with a CSA history who engage in SAC are almost always unaware of salient aspects of their SAC behavior. This fact provides an important clue to the dissociative quality that SAC has for them.

THE DISSOCIATIVE NATURE OF SAC

With remarkable frequency, throughout the process of discussing particular instances of SAC clients, information will come to light that may seem glaringly obvious but which never fully registered for the client despite innumerable instances of engaging in the behavior. What is most striking about the unrecognized components of the SAC pattern is that they often strongly contradict the client's previously held assumptions about the behavior. Consider, for example, the following vignettes from the treatment of SAC clients with histories of CSA:

> A woman in her early thirties had been sexually molested by an adult male baby sitter and by her brother in childhood. She reported engaging in many sexual contacts with strangers. She insisted that sex was intensely pleasurable to her and that this is what motivated these encounters. However, discussion of each particular sexual incident inevitably yielded an account of how disappointing, ungratifying, humiliating, or even physically painful the sexual activity had been. These descriptions often culminated in complaints about how sexually inept men were in general, and how they were only interested in their own pleasure.

> A man in his mid-twenties, who had been repeatedly sexually abused as a child by a woman friend of his mother, complained of a compulsive pattern of drinking and watching the dancers at strip clubs. He routinely promised himself to limit his time at the clubs to two or three hours, but found that up to eight hours elapsed before he could bring himself to leave. It had not occurred to him until he discussed this pattern in detail in therapy that it did not involve any explicit sexual gratification. He never purchased lap dances, never touched the dancers in any way, and after leaving the club would go home and fall asleep without masturbating or having sex with his wife.

A man in his early thirties had been sexually abused by his father throughout his early childhood, and had been raped by two men in his late teens. He compulsively picked up men for sex on the street and in various public places, but when asked to be more specific in describing these encounters revealed that the vast majority of the time he was unable to attain an erection or ejaculate. Despite this, it only gradually became clear to him during the course of therapy how little sexual pleasure he experienced both in his SAC contacts and in his sex life with his partner.

A woman in her late twenties who was molested as a child by her father worked as a dancer at a strip club. She insisted that she enjoyed her job, finding it emotionally and sexually exciting to have men watch her dance naked. Several months into therapy she found that she suddenly "came to" in the middle of performing at the club and was horrified as she became intensely aware of the men staring at her in a way that had never registered for her previously. She immediately stopped working at strip clubs.

A man in his late twenties who had been sexually molested by several different men during his childhood reported engaging in a large number of SAC behaviors every week. They included anonymous sexual contacts with men in public places, masturbating during anonymous phone calls, and masturbating to heterosexual pornography on the Internet. As specific instances of these behaviors were discussed in detail in treatment, it came to light that he was only able to achieve orgasm after long periods of time and with such intense amounts of friction that he sometimes experienced chaffing and occasionally produced bleeding.

As these vignettes illustrate, detailed examination of SAC routinely reveals evidence that the pattern of behavior includes a number of characteristics of which the client was unaware, and that often contradict her or his previous impression that the activity is pleasurable. These characteristics routinely include the following:

- Sexual dysfunction (e.g., routinely being unable to maintain an erection, ejaculate, or attain orgasm during SAC episodes);
- Explicitly aversive elements (e.g., extreme anxiety during certain phases of the SAC sequence, unwelcome physical discomfort or painful sensations accompanying the SAC behavior) of which the

client is *unaware* before discussing the specific SAC incidents in detail;

- Sexual numbing (e.g., engaging in sexual behavior while experiencing little or no sexual desire or arousal) of which the client is *unaware* before discussing the specific SAC incidents in detail;
- Ritualistic recapitulation in the SAC pattern of aspects of the CSA experience (e.g., repeating the same sexual activities that comprised the CSA, only choosing partners of SAC activities who resemble the CSA perpetrator physically or demographically) of which the client is *unaware* before discussing the specific SAC incidents in detail;
- Ritualistic adherence to limitations on sexual activity (e.g., rigid avoidance of activity involving penetration or of ejaculation during penetration);
- Difficulty remembering important aspects of the SAC incident even if it occurred just days or hours earlier;
- A subjective sense of being in a daze and of truncated awareness during the SAC incident;
- Absence of a sense of agency during SAC episodes (e.g., a sense of acting as if on "automatic pilot" or of feeling compelled to engage in the SAC behavior in a way that carries a sense of being coerced as if by someone else).

These characteristics suggest two major conclusions about SAC behavior among CSA survivors. One is that despite the appearance that the behavior is sexual in nature, SAC, at least among CSA survivors, is rarely unambiguously sexually fulfilling, and often includes frankly unpleasant or painful qualities. The other is that a number of observations strongly suggest the presence of dissociative factors. These phenomena include: lack of awareness of salient aspects of SAC patterns, despite repeated execution of these behaviors; poor recollection of SAC incidents even when they are recent; clouded awareness during SAC activity; and a sense that the behavior is occurring automatically and outside of conscious control. Empirical support for this inference is provided by a study that found that 20 out of 31 self-identified sex addicts in residential treatment assessed with the Structure Clinical Interview for Dissociative Disorders (SCID-D) were classified as having a dissociative disorder (Griffin-Shelley, Benjamin, & Benjamin, 1995). A relationship between SAC and dissociation in CSA survivors has also been noted in the clinical literature (Schwartz, Galperin, & Masters, 1995).

Indeed, one of the main ingredients of the SCAN-R procedure that seems to contribute to its effectiveness is that it breaks through the dissociative compartmentalization that seems to characterize SAC episodes among CSA survivors. This is part of the rationale for focusing the intervention on examining SAC behavior rather than directly exhorting the client to attempt to control or eliminate it. The almost universal gaps in recognition of major aspects of the SAC behavior pattern and their implications, along with the often-reported combination of cloudy awareness, poor recall, and lack of a sense of agency during episodes of SAC, strongly suggest that very little cognitive processing accompanies SAC.

In discussing the details of a number of SAC incidents over the course of treatment, the client is required to attend to, and to examine, what previously was occurring largely independently of cognitive processing. Each time SAC episodes are reviewed with the therapist in session, more cognitive appraisal becomes associated with them. In order to describe them to the therapist, the client is required to think about them in a more conscious, deliberate fashion than she or he had previously. When SAC behaviors are engaged in on subsequent occasions, it is not only with increased understanding attained by having examined them in treatment, but also with the awareness that they will later be revealed to the therapist. Repeatedly cycling between the two steps of interpersonal disclosure and appraisal of incidents of SAC with the therapist creates a cognitive bridge that pierces the dissociation that previously insulated SAC from other aspects of living.

OTHER COMPONENTS OF SAC TARGETED BY SCAN-R

Reduction of the dissociative aspect of SAC behavior is not the only reason why SCAN-R seems to be effective. The procedure reveals that participation in SAC behavior frequently elicits self-critical thinking and associated feelings such as shame, guilt, and low self-esteem among CSA survivors. Survivors often see their SAC activities as verification of the broader view they commonly hold of themselves as being wicked, repulsive, and undeserving of respect and esteem.

The SCAN-R procedure subtly and powerfully counteracts these perceptions and feelings. By calmly inquiring about the details of episodes of SAC behavior, the therapist inherently and powerfully demonstrates that these activities can be discussed and examined without censure or judgment. Talking about SAC with an accepting clinician who matter-of-factly inquires about specifics helps the client to become less judgmental about her or his own behavior and deconditions the anxiety experienced about these activities. As the patterns of SAC activity are analyzed, the client comes to understand that they are not driven by dark and perverse desires. Instead, clients usually come to the conclusion that their SAC patterns are triggered by circumstances that are particularly stressful for them and represent attempts to defuse the resulting distress.

Another common aspect of SAC behavior is that it is often secretive and is rarely discussed with others in any but the most general terms. Repeatedly talking about SAC experiences removes the secretiveness associated with it. This simultaneously helps to reduce dissociative compartmentalization of episodes of SAC, opening them up to a much greater level of cognitive processing than existed previously, and diminishing the anxiety and shame associated with them.

In many instances one factor that fuels SAC in CSA survivors is that it is an attempt to obtain the semblance of interpersonal closeness without taking the risks inherent in emotional intimacy. Revealing the very sensitive material comprising SAC activity to the clinician and feeling understood and accepted often stands in stark contrast to the relatively impersonal and alienating experience of SAC itself. Gradually, the SAC behavior becomes less firmly embedded in dissociative states. It is more clearly perceived and understood cognitively, and is recognized as not being sexually motivated and as largely sexually unfulfilling. It consequently carries progressively less negative self-appraisal and shame, and no longer operates in the shadows of secretiveness. As the patterning of the SAC behavior comes into focus, its occurrence can be anticipated in response to certain triggers and stressors. As the client becomes increasingly aware of the contrast between the detached quality of SAC episodes and the interpersonal attachment experienced in interaction with the therapist, the urge to engage in SAC behavior diminishes markedly. When the urge to participate in SAC behavior does arise, there is enough capacity for recognition of the presence of these impulses to exercise forethought about whether to act on them and to invoke relapse prevention strategies.

One of the more obvious reasons for the effectiveness of the SCAN-R procedure is that the more aware the client becomes of a SAC behavior's aversive and unfulfilling aspects, the less motivation there is to repeat the behavior. Simply put, the light cast on the activity by increasing cognitive awareness of its actual nature powerfully counteracts the perception that the SAC activity is "fun." Although this in itself may not entirely eliminate the pull to engage in SAC behavior, it usually does substantially reduce its intensity.

In the absence of awareness of the emotional or physical discomfort and lack of sexual pleasure or gratification associated with the SAC behavior, clients believe themselves to be hypersexual and sex-obsessed. As they come to realize that many if not all of the motivations that have been driving participation in SAC are non-sexual, this self-perception changes radically. In fact, as it becomes increasingly apparent how little sexual fulfillment and how much sexual numbness characterizes SAC behavior, some clients come to realize that rather than being hypersexual, they have really been severely limited in their capacity for experiencing intense sexual arousal and pleasure. As the desire to engage in SAC wanes, these clients become increasingly invested in learning to access the sexual pleasure and responsiveness that they now realize has been previously unavailable to them.

SCAN-R IN THE CONTEXT OF CONTEXTUAL THERAPY

Our impression in attempting to use SCAN-R as a stand-alone treatment is that it is much less likely to be effective when employed in this way than when incorporated into the larger framework comprising contextual therapy. It is not within the scope of this paper to provide an overview of contextual therapy in its entirety. However, we do believe it is important to understand why SCAN-R is likely to be ineffective when divorced from the rest of contextual treatment, and how the SCAN-R procedure is related to the conceptual framework that underlies this form of therapy.

At the core of a contextual conceptualization is the observation that many CSA survivors in clinical populations report an extensive history of childhood maltreatment, often by a number of perpetrators, which seems to be integrally related to the familial and social context in which they grew up. Whether or not CSA is committed by relatives, the family backgrounds in which such clients are reared often are characterized by low levels of cohesiveness, high levels of conflict, and, in general, markedly ineffective or inconsistent parenting (Gold, 2000). These factors interfere with the development of secure attachment, thwart the acquisition and mastery of fundamental knowledge and skills required for adequate daily functioning, and through parental modeling promote the acquisition of counter-productive coping strategies, such as substance abuse, aggressively lashing out at others, and self-harm. This perspective suggests that many of the difficulties of these clients are attributable not only to the CSA to which they were subjected, but to the family and social context in which they were reared. In fact, the emotional deprivation and unassertiveness that this type of family background often engenders may play an instrumental role in making these individuals particularly vulnerable to sexual molestation and other forms of abuse.

A crucial treatment implication of a contextual conceptualization is that while the trauma of CSA *disrupts* existing adaptive capacities, an ineffective family background *obstructs them from being acquired in the first place*. Trauma-focused treatment can *restore* abilities weakened by abuse, but obviously cannot *instill* capacities that were never adequately mastered. Contextual treatment, therefore, while it incorporates trauma-related interventions, is more broadly designed to promote the identification and remediation of gaps in adaptive functioning that may have been compounded by abuse, but which appear to be attributed to contextual factors more pervasive than discrete incidents of maltreatment. Consequently, contextual therapy consists of three primary components: (a) establishment of a collaborative therapeutic relationship to help foster development of secure attachment; (b) facilitation of client conceptualization of how abuse trauma and family environment have contributed to current difficulties; and (c) remediation of specific skills needed for effective daily functioning.

The SCAN-R procedure falls largely in the third of these categories. It is a relatively concrete technique designed to help the client reduce and eventually eliminate reliance on the largely ineffective coping strategy of SAC behavior, to replace that coping mechanism with more productive ones, and to subsequently develop the capacities for sexual responsiveness and fulfillment. However, when not integrated into a broader treatment framework including the relationship component, which helps address attachment difficulties, and the conceptual component, which provides a perspective that counteracts self-rejection and self-blame, SCAN-R is highly unlikely to be successful. (See Schwartz & Southern (1999) for a detailed discussion of the possible relationships between CSA, SAC and attachment deficits.) Other aspects of contextual treatment that increase the probability of positive outcomes in recovery from SAC are interventions aimed at the reduction of elevated levels of distress and dissociation before SCAN-R is implemented. In brief, SCAN-R should be considered part of a more comprehensive treatment program for survivors of prolonged childhood abuse who engage in SAC behavior, rather than a stand-alone intervention for SAC.

COMPARISON WITH OTHER SAC TREATMENT APPROACHES

The proposed treatment approaches for SAC have been wide-ranging, spanning psychopharmacological interventions (e.g., Kafka & Prentky, 1992; Stein et al., 1992; Suarez, O'Leary, Morgenstern, Allen, & Hollender, 2002), group therapy (e.g., Line & Cooper, 2002; Nerenberg, 2000; Quadland, 1985), cognitive behavioral therapy (e.g., Walch & Prejean, 2001), couples therapy (e.g., Manley, 1999; Sprenkle, 1987), family systems therapy (e.g., Corley & Alvarez, 1996), Gestalt therapy (Friedman, 1999), art therapy (Wilson, 1999) and integrated approaches (Schwartz & Masters, 1994). Despite these variations, however, most existing treatment models for SAC are built upon Twelve Step programs for alcohol dependency and other addictions or incorporate Twelve Step into a broader integrated program of treatment (see, e.g., Carnes, 1983; 1989; 1991; Earle & Crowe, 1990; Goodman, 1992; Pincu, 1989; Quadland, 1985). Carnes (1983; 1989; 1991) was instrumental in developing the notion that sexual compulsivity was similar to addiction to substances and in promoting the concept of sexual addiction. He helped raise awareness that substance abuse and other compulsive and addictive behaviors often co-occur, that it is not unusual to shift between multiple substance addictions and other compulsive behaviors, and that the Twelve Step model that has been employed for recovery from substance addictions can be applied to SAC. In some Twelve-Step-related approaches participation in Twelve Step groups is seen as primary, with psychotherapy playing a more or less adjunctive role. As Carnes (1989) puts it:

> Some [sex] addicts can recover simply by participating in a Twelve Step group–especially a strong one with a committed membership and accountability. In most cases, the additional help of a therapist is needed. (p. 230)

The concept of "unmanageability" in Twelve Step programs is very similar to the notion in contextual therapy that many survivors of prolonged CSA lack adequate resources to cope effectively with daily living. However, these two approaches make opposing assumptions about the cause and effect relationship between SAC and unmanageability. According to the Twelve Step addictions model, "life becomes unmanageable due to compulsive sexual behavior" (Carnes, 1989, p. 184) and as a result of other, co-existing addictive and compulsive patterns.

Therefore, in an addictions model, gaining control over SAC behavior is a precursor to learning to develop a more manageable lifestyle. In contrast, a contextual perspective suggests that, at least for prolonged CSA survivors, SAC develops, in part, in response to the unavailability of more effective means of coping. Consequently, in contextual therapy, the initial emphasis is on developing a more stable lifestyle; once significant progress is made toward this goal, then SAC is more directly targeted. In general, it is important to keep in mind that contextual therapy and SCAN-R were specifically developed for CSA survivors with SAC, and may be inappropriate for and ineffective with clients with SAC who do not have a CSA history.

CONCLUSIONS: CSA, SAC AND DISSOCIATION

We have reported here on our clinical observation that SAC patterns of behavior are especially prevalent among CSA survivors, especially male survivors. We also discuss clinical evidence obtained through the SCAN-R procedure that SAC in CSA survivors is often accompanied by dissociative characteristics and sexual dysfunction. Assuming that the validity and generalizability of these clinical observations are supported by empirical investigation, what may account for the relationship between CSA, SAC, dissociation and sexual dysfunction?

From a trauma-centered conceptual framework, SAC can be construed as a reenactment of the original CSA experiences. In some cases, there is compelling evidence for this. We have seen instances in which the SAC behaviors in which the client engages are rigidly confined to the same sex acts that comprised their CSA experiences, to partners that physically or demographically resemble the perpetrator(s) of their CSA, or to the setting or other circumstances in which their CSA took place. From this perspective, repeatedly engaging in SAC could be seen as an unwitting attempt to master the trauma of CSA. This explanation seems consistent with the dissociative features that often appear to accompany SAC behavior in survivors. Conceptualizing SAC as a reenactment of CSA would also account for the why SAC behaviors persist despite limitations in levels of sexual desire, arousal or fulfillment.

However, not all SAC behavior patterns manifested by CSA survivors resemble their CSA experiences. An additional explanation of SAC among CSA survivors is that it can at least in part be attributed to the various deficits in adaptation associated with growing up in an ineffective family context. From this perspective, dissociation can be understood as being related to insecure or disorganized attachment due to the lack of consistent availability and responsivity of caretakers. Lack of secure attachment, in turn, translates into disconnectedness from others, from one's own emotional experience, and from the immediate present, all of which interfere with the capacities for sexual responsiveness, emotional intimacy, and the integration of these two spheres of capacities.

Growing up in an interpersonal context in which emotional support, validation, and responsiveness are minimal, absent, or inconsistently available, instills a sense of being unlovable, undesirable, or even reprehensible in the developing child while simultaneously creating an intense yearning for affection and affirmation of worth (Gold, 2000). This combination of low self-esteem and emotional neediness leaves the child particularly vulnerable to sexual abuse and other forms of coercive control. When CSA does occur, it can leave such a child with the conviction that her or his only value to others is as an object of sexual interest. Consequently, sexual contact may come to be seen as one of the few routes to experiencing a sense of validation of self and of connection with others. For this reason, episodes of SAC are most likely to occur in response to distress (e.g., anxiety, loneliness, humiliation) and the resulting need for soothing and validation. It is often this objective, rather than sexual desire, that emerges in the SCAN-R procedure as the motivation for engaging in SAC behaviors.

Obviously, these two explanations, abuse reenactment and a poorly developed capacity for attachment, are not mutually exclusive. In actuality, one often finds evidence for the presence of both factors in the development and maintenance of SAC. In either case, dissociative disconnection from the immediacy of sexual experience can be understood as a major reason why SAC persists even though it may actually be sexually and emotionally unsatisfying or even aversive. Since it is carried out in the automatic, experientially detached manner that defines dissociative phenomena, recollection, recognition, and integration of the unsatisfactory nature of SAC is unlikely to occur. One of the major mechanisms via which SCAN-R appears to defuse the addictive/compulsive process is by helping the client to break through the dissociative barrier that isolates SAC experiences from focal cognitive awareness and processing. It is for this reason that we believe that recognition of the dissociative quality of SAC behavior is essential to adequately understanding it, and that targeting the dissociative elements of SAC behavior in treatment is crucial to disrupting it.

REFERENCES

Alexander, P.C. (1992). Application of attachment theory to the study of sexual abuse. *Journal of Consulting and Clinical Psychology*, *60*, 185-195.

Alexander, P.C. (1993). The differential effects of abuse characteristics and attachment in the prediction of long-term effects of sexual abuse. *Journal of Interpersonal Violence*, *8*, 346-362.

Allers, C.T., Benjack, K.J., White, J., & Rousey, J.T. (1993). HIV vulnerability and the survivor of sexual abuse. *Child Abuse and Neglect*, *17*, 291-298.

Anderson, G., Yasenik, L., & Ross, C.A. (1993). Dissociative experiences and disorders among women who identify themselves as sexual abuse survivors. *Child Abuse & Neglect*, *17*, 677-687.

Anderson, N., & Coleman, E. (1991). Childhood abuse and family sexual attitudes in sexually compulsive males: A comparison of three clinical groups. *American Journal of Preventative Psychiatry and Neurology*, *3*, 8-15.

Barth, R.J., & Kinder, B.N. (1987). The mislabeling of sexual impulsivity. *Journal of Sex and Marital Therapy*, *13*, 15-23.

Becker, J.V., Skinner, L.J., Abel, G., & Cichon, J. (1986). Level of postassault sexual functioning in rape and incest victims. *Archives of Sexual Behavior*, *15*, 37-49.

Bennett, E.K., & Kemper, K.J. (1994). Is abuse during childhood a risk factor for developing substance abuse problems as an adult? *Journal of Developmental & Behavioral Pediatrics*, *15*, 426-429.

Briere, J.N., & Elliott, D.M. (1994). Immediate and long-term impacts of child sexual abuse. *The Future of Children*, *4*, 54-69.

Briere, J., Evans, D., Runtz, M., & Wall, T. (1988). Symptomology in men who were molested as children: A comparison study. *American Journal of Orthopsychiatry*, *58*, 457-461.

Briere, J., & Runtz, M. (1987). Post sexual abuse trauma: Data and implications for clinical practice. *Journal of Interpersonal Violence*, *2*, 367- 379.

Briere, J., & Runtz, M. (1990). Differential adult symptomatology associated with three types of child abuse histories. *Child Abuse & Neglect*, *14*, 357-364.

Browne, A., & Finkelhor, D. (1986). Impact of sexual abuse: A review of the research. *Psychological Bulletin*, *99*, 66-77.

Browning, C.R., & Laumann, E.O. (1997). Sexual contact between children and adults: A life course perspective. *American Sociological Review*, *62*, 540-560.

Butts, J.D. (1992). The relationship between sexual addiction and sexual dysfunction. *Journal of Health Care for the Poor and Underserved*, *3*, 128-135.

Carnes, P. (1983). *Out of the shadows: Understanding sexual addiction*. Minneapolis, MN: CompCare Publishers.

Carnes, P. (1989). *Contrary to love: Helping the sex addict*. Minneapolis, MN: CompCare Publishers.

Carnes, P. (1991). *Don't call it love: Recovery from sexual addiction*. New York, NY: Bantam.

Carnes, P.J., & Delmonico, D.L. (1996). Childhood abuse and multiple addictions: Research findings in a sample of self-identified sexual addicts. *Sexual Addiction & Compulsivity*, *3*, 258-268.

Cavaiola, A.A., & Schiff, M. (1988). Behavioral sequelae of physical and/or sexual abuse in adolescents. *Child Abuse & Neglect*, *12*, 181-188.

Chu, J.A., & Dill, D.L. (1990). Dissociative symptoms in relation to childhood physical and sexual abuse. *American Journal of Psychiatry*, *147*, 887-892.

Coleman, E. (1992). Is your patient suffering from compulsive sexual behavior? *Psychiatric Annals*, *22*, 320-325.

Corley, M.D., & Alvarez, M. (1996). Including children and family in the treatment of individuals with compulsive and addictive disorders. *Sexual Addiction & Compulsivity*, *3*, 69-84.

Courtois, C.A. (1988). *Healing the incest wound: Adult survivors in therapy*. New York: W. W. Norton.

de Groot, J., & Rodin, G.M. (1999). The relationship between eating disorders and childhood trauma. *Psychiatric Annals*, *29*, 225-229.

Dhaliwal, G.K., Gauzas, L., Antonowicz, D.H., & Ross, R.R. (1996). Adult male survivors of childhood sexual abuse: Prevalence, sexual abuse characteristics, and long term effects. *Clinical Psychology Review*, *16*, 619-639.

Dimock, P.T. (1988). Adult males sexually abused as children: Characteristics and implications for treatment. *Journal of Interpersonal Violence*, *3*, 203-221.

Earle, R.H., & Crow, G.M. (1990). Sexual addiction: Understanding and treating the phenomenon. *Contemporary Family Therapy*, *12*, 89-104.

Fallon, P., & Wonderlich, S.A. (1997). Sexual abuse and other forms of trauma. In D.M. Garner & P.E. Garfinkel (Eds.), *Handbook of treatment for eating disorders* (pp. 394-414). New York: Guilford Press.

Finkelhor, D. (1990). Early and long-term effects of child sexual abuse: An update. *Professional Psychology: Research and Practice*, *21*, 325-330.

Fischer, B. (1995). Sexual addiction revisited. *The Addictions Newsletter*, *2*(3), 5, 27.

Friedman, H.R. (1999). A Gestalt approach to sexual compulsivity. *Sexual Addiction & Compulsivity*, *6*, 63-75.

Freyd, J.J. (1996). *Betrayal trauma: The logic of forgetting child abuse*. Cambridge, MA: Harvard University Press.

Gill, M., & Tutty, L. (1999). Male survivors of childhood sexual abuse: A qualitative study and issues for clinical consideration. *Journal of Childhood Sexual Abuse*, *17*(3), 19-33.

Gold, S.N. (2000). *Not trauma alone: Therapy for child abuse survivors in family and social context*. Philadelphia, PA: Brunner Routledge.

Gold, S.N. (in press). Recovery of people, not memories. *Journal of Child Sexual Abuse*.

Gold, S.N., & Heffner, C.L. (1998). Sexual addiction: Many conceptions, minimal data. *Clinical Psychology Review*, *18*, 367-381.

Goodman, A. (1992). Sexual addiction: Designation and treatment. *Journal of Sex and Marital Therapy*, *18*, 303-314.

Goodman, A. (1993). Diagnosis and treatment of sexual addiction. *Journal of Sex and Marital Therapy*, *19*, 225-251.

Griffin-Shelley, E., Benjamin, L., & Benjamin, R. (1995). Sex addiction and dissociation. *Sexual Addiction & Compulsivity*, *2*(4), 295-306.

Herman, J.L. (1992). *Trauma and recovery: The aftermath of violence–from domestic abuse to political terror*. New York: Basic Books.

Herman, J.L., Perry, J.C., & van der Kolk, B.A. (1989). Childhood trauma in borderline personality disorder. *American Journal of Psychiatry, 146*, 490-495.

Hunter, M., & Struve, J. (1998). Challenging the taboo: Support for the ethical use of touch in psychotherapy with sexually compulsive/addicted clients. *Sexual Addiction & Compulsivity, 5*, 141-148.

Kafka, M.P., & Prentky, R. (1992). Fluoxetine treatment of nonparaphilic sexual addiction and paraphilias in men. *Journal of Clinical Psychiatry, 53*, 351-358.

Kluft, R.P. (Ed.). (1990). *Incest-related syndromes of adult psychopathology*. Washington, DC: American Psychiatric Press.

Levin M.P., & Troiden, R.R. (1988). The myth of sexual compulsivity. *The Journal of Sex Research, 25*, 347-363.

Line, B.Y., & Cooper, A. (2002). Group therapy: Essential component for success with sexually acting out problems among men. *Sexual addiction & compulsivity, 9*, 15-32.

Lipschitz, D.S., Winegar, R.K., Nicolauou, A.L., Hartnick, E., Wolfson, M., & Southwich, S.M. (1999). Perceived abuse and neglect as risk factors for suicidal behavior in adolescent inpatients. *Journal of Nervous and Mental Disease, 187*, 32-39

Mackey, T.F., Hacker, S.S., Weissfeld, L.A., Ambrose, N.C., Fisher, M.G., & Zobel, D.L. (1991). Comparative effects of sexual assault on sexual functioning of child sexual abuse survivors and others. *Issues in Mental Health Nursing, 12*, 89-112.

Maltz, W. (1988). Identifying and treating the sexual repercussions of incest: A couples therapy approach. *Journal of Sex & Marital Therapy, 14*, 142-170.

Maltz, W. (1991). *The sexual healing journey: A guide for survivors of sexual abuse*. New York, NY: Harper Collins.

Maltz, W., & Holman, B. (1987). *Incest and sexuality: A guide to understanding and healing*. Lexington, MA: Lexington Books.

Manley, G. (1999). Treating chronic sexual dysfunction in couples recovering from sex addiction and sex coaddiction. *Sexual Addiction & Compulsivity, 6*, 111-124.

McCarthy, B. (1994). Sexually compulsive men and inhibited sexual desire. *Journal of Sex & Marital Therapy, 20*, 200-209.

McCauley, J., Kern, D.E., Koladner, K., Dill, L., Schroeder, A.E., DeChant, H.K., Ryden, J., Derogatis, L.R., & Bass, E.B. (1997). Clinical characteristics of women with a history of childhood abuse: Unhealed wounds. *Journal of the American Medical Association, 277*, 1362-1368.

Mullen, P.E., Martin, J.L., Anderson, J.C., Romans, S.E., & Herbison, G.P. (1996). The long-term impact of the physical, emotional, and sexual abuse of children: A community study. *Child Abuse & Neglect, 20*, 7-21.

Nerenberg, A. (2000). The value of group psychotherapy for sexual addicts in a residential setting. *Sexual Addiction & Compulsivity, 7*, 197-209.

Nijman, H.L.I., Dautzenberg, M., Merkelback, H.L.G.J., Jung, P., Wessel, I., & Campo, J. (1999). Self-mutilating behavior of psychiatric inpatients. *European Psychiatry, 14*, 4-10.

Perry, J.C., Herman, J.L., van der Kolk, B.A., & Holk, L.A. (1990). Psychotherapy and psychological trauma in borderline personality disorder. *Psychiatric Annals, 20*, 33-43.

Pincu, L. (1989). Sexual compulsivity in gay men: Controversy and treatment. *Journal of Counseling and Development, 68*, 63-66.

Quadland, M.C. (1985). Compulsive sexual behavior: Definitions of a problem and an approach to treatment. *Journal of Sex & Marital Therapy, 11*, 121-132.

Rodriguez, N., Ryan, S.W., Rowan, A.B., & Foy, D.W. (1996). Posttraumatic stress disorder in a clinical sample of adult's survivors of childhood sexual abuse. *Child Abuse & Neglect, 20*, 943-952.

Rowan, A.B., & Foy, D.W. (1993). Posttraumatic stress disorder in child sexual abuse survivors: A literature review. *Journal of Traumatic Stress, 6*, 3-20.

Schwartz, M.F., Galperin, L.D., & Masters, W.H. (1995). Dissociation and treatment of compulsive reenactment of trauma: Sexual compulsivity. In M. Hunter (Ed.), *Adult survivors of sexual abuse: Treatment innovations* (pp. 42-55). Thousand Oaks, CA: Sage.

Schwartz, M.F., & Masters, W.H. (1994). Integration of trauma-based, cognitive, behavioral, systematic and addiction approaches for treatment of hypersexual pair-bonding disorder. *Sexual Addiction & Compulsivity, 1*, 57-76.

Schwartz, M.F., & Southern, S. (1999). Manifestations of damaged development of the human affectional systems and developmentally based psychotherapies. *Sexual Addiction & Compulsivity, 6*, 163-175.

Schwartz, M.F., & Southern, S. (2000). Compulsive cybersex: The new tearoom. Sexual *Addiction and Compulsivity, 7*, 127-144.

Spak, L., Spak, F., & Allebeck, P. (1997). Factors in childhood and youth predicting alcohol dependence and abuse in Swedish women: Findings from a general population study. *Alcohol & Alcoholism, 32*, 267-274.

Sprenkle, D.H. (1987). Treating a sex addict through marital therapy. *Family Relations: Journal of Applied Family & Child Studies, 36*, 11-14.

Stein, D.J., Hollander, E., Anthony, D.T., Schneider, F.R., Fallon, B.A., Liebowitz, M.R., & Klein, D.F. (1992). Serotonergic medications for sexual obsessions, sexual addictions, and paraphilias. *Journal of Clinical Psychiatry, 53*, 267-271.

Suarez, T., O'Leary, A., Morgenstern, J., Allen, A., & Hollander, E. (2002). Selective serotonin reuptake inhibitors as a treatment for sexual compulsivity. In A. O'Leary (Ed.), *Beyond condoms: Alternative approaches to HIV prevention* (pp. 199-200). New York: Plenum.

Tedesco, A., & Bola, J.R. (1997). A pilot study of the relationship between childhood sexual abuse and compulsive sexual behaviors in adults. *Sexual Addiction and Compulsivity, 4*, 147-157.

Tsai, M., Feldman-Summers, S., & Edgar, M. (1979). Child molestation: Variables related to differential impacts on psychosexual functioning in adult women. *Journal of Abnormal Psychology, 88*, 407-417.

Walch, S.E., & Prejean, J. (2001). Reducing HIV risk from compulsive sexual behavior using cognitive behavioral therapy within a harm reduction framework: A case example. *Sexual Addiction & Compulsivity, 8*, 113-128.

Walser, R.D., & Kern, J.M. (1996). Relationships among childhood sexual abuse, sex guilt, and sexual behavior in adult clinical samples. *Journal of Sex Research, 33*, 321-326.

Westerlund, E. (1983). Counseling women with histories of incest. *Women & Therapy*, *2*, 17-31.

Westerlund, E. (1992). *Women's sexuality after childhood incest*. New York, NY: W.W. Norton & Co.

Whitfield, C.L. (1998). Internal evidence and corroboration of traumatic memories of child sexual abuse with addictive disorders. *Sexual Addiction and Compulsivity*, *4*, 269-292.

Wilsnack, S.C., Vogeltanz, N.D., Klassen, A.D., & Harris, T. R. (1997). Childhood sexual abuse and women's substance abuse: National survey findings. *Journal of Studies on Alcohol*, *58*, 264-271.

Wilson, M. (1999). Art therapy with the invisible sex addict. *Art Therapy*, *16*, 7-16.

Some Considerations About Sexual Abuse and Children with Sexual Behavior Problems

Toni Cavanagh Johnson, PhD

SUMMARY. In the mid 1980s treatment programs for children twelve years and younger who molested other children began to appear. There was little known about these children and there were numerous misconceptions about this population. It was believed that the primary etiological factor in the development of this behavior was previous hands-on sexual abuse to the child. It was also believed that a majority of sexually abused children would engage in problematic sexual behaviors and that it was quite likely that they would go on to molest others. In the intervening years a great deal has been learned about children who molest. The diversity of reasons for the development of problematic sexual behavior has been researched. Another important finding is that there is a range of disturbed sexual behaviors in children. This is important as there has been an overidentification of children who engage in problematic sexual behaviors as children who are molesting. A continuum of sexual behaviors in children is described which delineates three groups of children who engage in problematic sexual behavior, only one of which is molesting other children. With this understanding professionals can distinguish

---

Toni Cavanagh Johnson is in the independent practice of clinical psychology, South Pasadena, CA

Address correspondence to: Toni Cavanagh Johnson, PhD, Licensed Clinical Psychologist PSY 9532, 1101 Fremont Avenue, Suite 101, South Pasadena, CA 91030 (E-mail: TcavJohn@aol.com).

[Haworth co-indexing entry note]: "Some Considerations About Sexual Abuse and Children with Sexual Behavior Problems." Johnson, Toni Cavanagh. Co-published simultaneously in *Journal of Trauma & Dissociation* (The Haworth Medical Press, an imprint of The Haworth Press, Inc.) Vol. 3, No. 4, 2002, pp. 83-105; and: *Trauma and Sexuality: The Effects of Childhood Sexual, Physical, and Emotional Abuse on Sexuality Identity and Behavior* (ed: James A. Chu, and Elizabeth S. Bowman) The Haworth Medical Press, an imprint of The Haworth Press, Inc., 2002, pp. 83-105. Single or multiple copies of this article are available for a fee from The Haworth Document Delivery Service [1-800-HAWORTH, 9:00 a.m. - 5:00 p.m. (EST). E-mail address: getinfo@haworthpressinc.com].

between children who engage in natural and healthy sexual behaviors, sexually-reactive behaviors, extensive but mutual sexual behaviors, and children who molest. This assists in more accurate assessment and treatment planning in an era in which children can be placed on sex offender registries and potentially be subject to community notification.

KEYWORDS. Children, child sexual abuse, children with sexual behavior problems, child dissociative disorders

In 1985, the first treatment program designed exclusively to treat children (twelve years and younger) who sexually molest other children and their families opened its doors at Children's Institute International in Los Angeles. There was very little understanding at that time about this special population of children.

- What are the etiological factors behind this behavior?
- Are all children who molest victims of sexual abuse?
- How many victims of sexual abuse will molest other children?
- How many children who sexually abuse other children are there?
- Are all children who are engaging in problematic sexual behaviors molesting other children?
- How should we define molesting behavior in children?
- What is natural and healthy sexual behavior in children and how does this differ from molesting?

These and many more questions were of immediate concern to the program as it sought to develop treatment tailored to an understanding of the children and their families.

ARE ALL CHILDREN WHO MOLEST VICTIMS OF SEXUAL ABUSE?

At the inception there was a belief that the major etiological factor for the molesting behavior by the children was that they had been sexually abuse. This belief was based on the incorrect notion that virtually all adult sex offenders had been sexually abused, and that the cause for their sexual offending was having been sexually abused (Hanson & Slater, 1988; Murphy & Peters, 1992). As more children who molested were brought into treatment, it was discovered that many did not talk about being sexually abused. As most of the children were boys, a belief developed that the reason more hands-on sexual abuse was not being found in the histories of the children was due to it being difficult for boys to disclose sexual abuse.

In the mid 1980s several articles were published about children who molested other children. In a sample of 14 boys and four girls, Friedrich and Luecke (1988) found that 75% of the "sexually-aggressive" boys and 100% of the "sexually-aggressive" girls had been sexually abused. In a sample of 47 boys, Johnson (1988) found that overall 50% of the children who molested had been sexually abused, with 72% of the 4-6 year olds, 42% of the 7-10 year olds, and 35% of the children between 11-12 years old being sexually abused. Virtually all of the boys had sustained pervasive harsh physical punishment. Forty-six percent (46%) of the victims of these boys were siblings, 18% were cousins, 16% were schoolmates and six percent were foster siblings. In an article on 13 girls who molest, Johnson (1989) found that all of the girls had been sexually abused and they had sustained pervasive harsh physical punishment. Of the first victims of the girls, 54% were siblings, 23% were cousins, and 23%were friends.

While the samples of children who molest were small, the lower than expected incidence of sexual abuse in boys was corroborated by information gathered on adult sex offenders. Murphy and Peters (1992) wrote, "There is a good deal of clinical lore that a history of being sexually victimized is predominant in the backgrounds of sex offenders. However, there are a number of problems when extrapolating the clinical lore to the legal arena. First, one must realize that estimates currently suggest that somewhere between 1 in 9 children to 1 in 10 young males will be sexually abused before the age of 18 (Finkelhor, Hotaling, Lewis, & Smith, 1990). The vast majority of these children do not grow up to be sex offenders and therefore one could not classify someone as a sex offender based on the fact that they have been sexually abused. In addition, (Hanson & Slater, 1988) reviewed data on 1,717 offenders included in 18 different studies. They found that the average rate of sexual abuse across studies was 28%" (pp. 33).

Although the empirical literature indicated that not all children who molest other children were themselves victims of sexual abuse, this belief has persisted in the minds of the general public, and in some police, child protective service workers and mental health professionals (Friedrich & Chaffin, 2000). It is important to counteract this belief in professionals, as some may influence children who molest to make a disclosure of sexual abuse when there has been none. Children may believe that there is only one acceptable explanation for their molesting behavior and move to satisfy the belief of the therapist by fabricating a history of sexual abuse. It is also important that children themselves do not believe that, if they were molested, this is the sole reason for their molesting behavior. This could act as a reason, justification, or a lessening of resolve to curtail sexually aggressive feelings and behaviors. It could also make them feel less competent to cease from engaging in such behaviors. This belief can also dishearten parents who may feel that if their children have been sexually abused that they are destined to engage in aggressive sexual behavior.

The belief that sexually abused children will molest others has had the effect on many in the general public of seeing child sexual abuse victims as a potential threat to their children. Children who have been sexually abused are unjustifiably seen as at substantial risk to molest others (Friedrich & Chaffin 2000). In schools, foster homes and even in the child's biological home, sexual behavior by a sexually abused child is often seen as far more disturbed than the same sexual behavior by a child who has not been sexually abused.

Understanding the etiological factors for children to molest other children is still in its infancy. Much work remains to be done. Several studies funded by the National Center on Child Abuse and Neglect found similar factors as in the Johnson (1988, 1989) and Friedrich and Luecke (1988) studies (Bonner, 1998; Gray, 1996; Gray, Busconi, Houchens, & Pithers, 1997; Gray, Pithers, Busconi, & Houchens, 1999; Pithers, Gray, Busconi, & Houchens, 1998a, 1998b). The Child Sexual Behavior Checklist (Johnson, 1998) was developed to evaluate the sexual behaviors of the children who have been identified as in need of therapy for sexual behavior problems. Question 17 in Part III asks if the child witnessed violence between people he or she knows. Our unpublished data shows that respondents consistently report that children who molest have witnessed violence between their parents or caretakers. It is possible that some children who live in homes with domestic violence believe that sex and aggression are complementary. Children who live in homes with partner violence often hear intense arguments in which one parent accuses the other of sexual misconduct, attempts to control all of the behaviors of that parent and emotionally and/or physically hurts the other parent as a payback for the alleged or real infidelity.

Children hear angry sexual language and witness violent interactions between parental figures, in which one parent violates the other's sexual rights. Children do not learn that sex is an expression of love between two people. Rather, constant fighting and jealousy by parents related to sex teaches the children that people use sex to hurt other people and that violence in relation to sex is natural. When sex might possibly appear to be a caring act is generally after violence has occurred. This pairing may also cause confusion for the child's developing template for sexual relationships. In the homes of children who molest, the children are very aware of the trauma and violence in the parents'/caretakers' lives and often become part of the drama as one or the other parent pulls them in as an ally or a scapegoat.

HOW MANY VICTIMS OF SEXUAL ABUSE WILL MOLEST OTHER CHILDREN?

The belief that sexual abuse was the major etiological factor for sexually abusive behavior in children spawned the alternate belief that children who were sexually abused were likely to sexually abuse other children. This belief has persisted, in spite of literature since 1987 to the contrary. As Kaufman and Zigler (1987) have observed:

> The findings of the different investigations are not easily integrated because of their methodological variations. Nonetheless, the best estimate of intergenerational transmission appears to be 30% plus or minus 5%. This suggests that approximately one-third of all individuals who were physically abused, sexually abused, or extremely neglected will subject their offspring to one of these forms of maltreatment, while the remaining two-thirds will provide adequate care for their children. The rate of abuse among individuals with a history of abuse (30 plus or minus 5%) is approximately six times higher than the base rate for abuse in the general population (5%).
>
> Being maltreated as a child puts one at risk for becoming abusive but the path between these two points is far from direct or inevitable. In the past, unqualified acceptance of the intergenerational hypothesis has had many negative consequences. Adults who were maltreated have been told so many times that they will abuse their children that for some it has become a self-fulfilling prophecy. Many who have broken the cycle are left feeling like

> walking time bombs. In addition, persistent acceptance of this belief has impeded progress in understanding the etiology of abuse and led to misguided judicial and social policy interventions. The time has come for the intergenerational myth to be put aside and for researchers to cease asking, "Do abused children become abusive parents?" and ask, instead, "Under what conditions is the transmission of abuse most likely to occur." (p. 192)

Research on sexually abused children does not show that the majority of sexually abused children will engage in worrisome sexual behaviors, much less sexually abusive behaviors. In a meta analysis of studies of sexually abused children Kendall-Tackett, Williams, and Finkelhor (1993) noted: "Across six studies of sexually abused preschoolers (the children most likely to manifest such symptoms) an average of 35% exhibited sexualized behavior" (p. 170). Friedrich, Gramsch, and Damon (1992), using an instrument specially designed to measure a wide range of sexual behaviors, detected a somewhat higher percentage. But across all sexually abused children it may be only a half of all victims who engage in any type of sexual behavior when younger than 12. The lowest estimate was 7% based on a very large study, including many well functioning older children (Conte & Schuerman, 1987).

Johnson (1998) estimated that less than .5 % of sexually abused children would go on to sexually abuse other children during childhood. In fact, specialized residential treatment programs for children who molest are generally unable to find sufficient numbers of children with the severest level of sexual behavior problem to fill up their beds (Johnson, 1998). Unable to fill all of their beds with children who sexually offend, these facilities accept children with a lesser degree of sexual problems. This can present a danger to children who are sexualized but who are not offending (see below, A Continuum of Sexual Behaviors).

The belief that if a child were sexually abused, the child would go on to abuse other children has been especially strong when a child, particularly a boy, has been sexually abused in a particularly cruel manner and for an extended amount of time. This can have exceptionally negative and unfair effects on the sexually abused and traumatized child as illustrated in the following clinical vignette.

> Enrique's early life while financially poor, was enriched by his mother's love. His recollections of his mother are very fond. He remembers no turmoil or trouble at any time when they lived together. He recalls spending a great deal of time at amusement

parks. He wants to preserve this idealized view of his mother as it is all he has of his past.

His mother lived on and off with his birth father who was physically abusive to her and had many extramarital affairs. Enrique's father left before he was four. He has no recollection of his father–no physical or mental picture of him.

Enrique's mother remarried when he was six years old. This marriage was also very violent and abusive. His mother was raped and physically battered repeatedly by her second husband. After having two children, she left him. In order to get money from the second husband to care for her three children, she complied with the husband's demand that Enrique go over to his house when he requested. During these visits to his stepfather's home, Enrique was locked in a room, blindfolded, and chained to a bed. The stepfather and other men sodomized Enrique and forced him into oral/genital contact. If he told his mother, Enrique was fearful for his mother's life and that his stepfather would sexually abuse his brothers. The stepfather reinforced these threats every time he dropped Enrique home.

By chance, Enrique's stepfather was stopped for a traffic violation. Pornographic pictures of Enrique being sodomized and fellated by the father and other men were found in his possession. Enrique and his two brothers were removed from his mother due to lack of protection and put in foster care. Due to the social worker's concern that Enrique would molest his brothers because he had been sexually abused, they were separated into different foster homes. After his stepfather was convicted of sexual assault and sent to prison, his mother absconded. Enrique never heard from her again. Lost and alone, his behavior escalated into rages and destruction of property. The staff in the residential facility feared that he would sexually victimize other boys in the facility and watched him diligently. Any hint of physical contact, that was vaguely suspicious, got strong reprimands from the staff. They made it clear that they did not trust him to be close to any of the children, due to "his history."

In the course of the treatment it became evident that Enrique's rages and destructive behaviors exploded when he felt trapped, or unloved and misunderstood. These two situations related directly to traumatic events and memories in his earlier life. In school situations, if the teacher demanded that he finish his work, and would not allow him to take a break or take a time out, but made him sit at his desk, Enrique would hear the voice of his stepfather and see his face. In a dissociated state, he would see black and go into a rage. Unaware of where he actually was, he would lash out and try to run away, sometimes throwing things. This feeling of being trapped and unable to move, catapulted him back to the sexual abuse, locked in the room, blindfolded and chained. When the staff tried to restrain him, he would struggle violently to get away. He never hurt any staff.

His feeling of absolute emotional devastation at the disappearance of his mother created overwhelming feelings in him that he couldn't tolerate and would frequently dissociate. At other times, when he experienced these feelings of loss he would externalize the terrifying feelings and blame her loss on the staff. In his thinking, if he hadn't been taken away from her and placed in residential treatment, his mother never would have left him; therefore it was Child Protective Services and the staff who sent his mother away. He could not emotionally tolerate alternative explanations for her disappearance. This irrational thought would pervade his thinking and he would become argumentative. He would then engage staff in interminable circular verbal altercations about his current behavior that were without foundation, and sometimes destroy property. On these occasions he was in a dissociated state and had no control of himself and little recollection of the events until the next day.

Enrique rarely argued intensely with the female staff, and always sought out one female staff person to relate to in a positive manner. Throughout his time in out-of-home care he found a "protective female" staff to whom he could talk and go to after his rages. He would relate to this staff person as if she were his mother. There were no sexual overtones attached. Unfortunately, due to the highly fluid nature of residential staff, Enrique would frequently become attached to a female staff who would leave for a higher paying position. Each of these losses further catapulted Enrique into despair and dissociation of the devastating feelings. While a protective female staff person fulfilled some of his needs for nurturing, she could rarely stop his rages. In fact, staff would say that many times he seemed to see and hear no one.

When Enrique began to understand the trauma-related nature of his thoughts and feelings and was able to talk about his mother, his abuse and his fears, he needed to dissociate less. However, he continued to have major problems in interactions with staff who triggered memories of his abuse. After his dissociative process was diagnosed and he agreed that his therapist could talk with him and the staff together to develop methods to assist him, his dissociative states gradually diminished. Enrique was able to use methods to ground himself in the present, internally say and think soothing thoughts, while the staff verbally assisted him to stay present and know what was happening and that there was no present danger and then direct him to a person to help him. With this, and the development of strong and permanent attachments, the rages abated totally.

Unfortunately, the staff at his facility continued to believe that he would sexually abuse someone due to the severity of his abuse. There were no reported aggressive sexual thoughts or desires on Enrique's part towards either adults or children. At age 15 Enrique began a relationship with a same age girl. At six months into the relationship there were no sexual problems. He was aware of his strong desire for a relationship to replace his parents and of the abandonment he may feel, if the relationship ends with the girl leaving him. He continued to monitor his sexual feelings, thoughts and behaviors for any confusion, aggressive or submissive trends.

A CONTINUUM OF SEXUAL BEHAVIORS

An additional complication that emerges when working with children with sexual behavior problems is defining when the sexual behavior is abusive and when it is less serious and not intended to harm, but is clearly beyond what can be considered within the normal and healthy range.

In a series of papers, I have described a continuum of sexual behaviors in children (Johnson, 1988, 1999, 2000). Along this continuum, four groups were identified. One group consists of children who engage in *natural and healthy sexual behaviors*. The other three groups consist of children with sexual behavior problems. These three groups are defined as: *sexually-reactive children*, *children who engage in extensive, mutual sexual behaviors*, and *children who molest other children*. I believe it is essential to differentiate between the three groups because the treatment needs and the "systems" interventions are different. This differentiation is also essential in making certain that children with less serious sexual behaviors are not misidentified as children who molest.

Natural and Healthy Sexual Behaviors

Natural and healthy sexual exploration during childhood is an information-gathering process in which young people explore each other's bodies by looking and touching ("playing doctor") as well as by exploring gender roles and behaviors ("playing house"). Children involved in healthy sexual play are of similar age, size, and developmental status and participate on a voluntary basis.

When siblings engage in mutual sexual exploration, most sexual play is between children who have an ongoing, mutually enjoyable play and/or school friendship. Their sexual behaviors are limited in type and frequency and occur at several periods of their young lives. Children's interest in sex and sexuality is balanced by their curiosity about other aspects of their lives. Healthy sexual exploration may result in embarrassment but does not usually result in deep feelings of anger, shame, fear, or anxiety. If children are discovered in sexual exploration and instructed to stop, the behavior generally diminishes, at least in the view of adults. Children's feelings regarding their sexual behavior are generally light-hearted and spontaneous. Children usually experience pleasurable sensations from genital touching. Some children experience sexual arousal while some children experience orgasm. Sexual arousal and orgasm are reported more frequently in older children entering puberty (Johnson, 1988, 1999, 2000).

Sexually-Reactive Children

These children may engage in self-stimulating behaviors and/or sexual behaviors with other children and, sometimes, with adults. This type of sexual behavior is generally in response to environmental cues that are overly stimulating or reminiscent of previous abuse or to feelings that reawaken other traumatic or painful memories. Many of these children have lived in sexually overwhelming environments in which they have not been shielded from adult or adolescent sexuality.

These children engage in sexual behavior is a way of coping with overwhelming feelings of which they cannot make sense. Hiding the sexual behaviors or finding friends to engage in the behaviors in private may be less possible for these children as the behaviors may be compulsively used for tension-release. This type of sexual behavior is often not within the full conscious control of the child. In some situations, children are trying to make sense of something sexual done to them by doing it to someone else. They do not coerce others into sexual behaviors but act out their confusion on others in an attempt to reduce anxiety and confused sensations and feelings. Many do not understand their own or others' rights to privacy or physical space integrity. While there is no intent to hurt others, receiving sexual behaviors can be confusing for the other person and feel like a violation or abuse (Johnson, 1988, 1999, 2000).

In the following vignette, the problem with differentiating between sexually abusive and sexually-reactive behavior is illustrated. Additionally, the confusion of environmentally induced confusion rather than hands-on sexual abuse to the child is portrayed.

> Tanya was born to a 19-year old drug-addicted mother. Her mother had no knowledge who the father was. Throughout Tanya's early life she lived with her mother in different motel rooms. During this time Tanya took care of her mother, soothing her when she was distraught, talking to her when she wanted to talk, and being quiet when she didn't want her to talk. To get food and drugs Tanya's mother engaged in sexual relations with a very wide variety of men. While her mother engaged in sexual activity with the men, Tanya would look on. Over the course of these early years, Tanya called 911 on three separate occasions when her mother had been badly beaten up by one of the men.
>
> During Tanya's first three and a half years of life her mother had two other children. Tanya did her best to help care for the littler children. After the first two 911 calls, the children stayed with their maternal grandmother who was alcoholic while their mother recuperated. After the third 911 call, the Child Protective Services placed all three children in foster care and identified the mother's pattern of behavior to the court. After this the mother disappeared for over a year and returned in a very weakened physical condition with severe liver damage.
>
> Tanya and her brother, Paul, were placed in a foster home in which the prospective foster parents had said that they would not accept children who had been sexually abused. The infant was placed in a different foster home. As there were no indications that the children had been sexually abused, Tanya and Paul moved into this foster home. Within three months of moving into the foster home, Tanya began to masturbate. The masturbation increased to the point that she was humping and rubbing her genitals in a rhythmic fashion almost everywhere. She would use the foster father's leg, the leg of the dining room table, the arms of the sofas, and

stuffed animals. In another few months she started to suck on the neck of the foster father, she touched the male social worker on the upper thigh, moving her hand toward his genitals.

Approximately six months into the placement Tanya was found humping her little brother, Paul, who was a year younger than her. The initial reaction of the social worker was to remove Tanya, saying that she was molesting her brother. However, Tanya's behavior was more akin to that of sexually-reactive children than children who molest. She liked her brother, and her humping of her brother was exactly what she had watched her mother do for years when the door to the bedroom was open. Her brother yelled to the foster parents to get her off of him. There was no force or coercion, no threats or intent to harm. Her brother said she just got on top of him and started humping. Since this author had just started providing service to Tanya, I requested that she not be removed but that we work with both children to decrease the sexual behavior and understand the source of the premature sexual activity.

The foster mother believed that Tanya had to have been sexually abused. While the possibility that Tanya was sexually abused in the situation in which she lived for her first four years of life were high, Tanya had no conscious recollection of having been touched in a sexual manner by any of the men who came into her mother's life. What did emerge in the course of the therapy were certain traumatic memories that precipitated Tanya into the sexual behaviors. Some triggers for the behavior were external to her and could be identified by others. Hearing any siren, whether it be police, fire, or ambulance, as well as hearing arguing between adults, or even minor disagreements, triggered her to sexual behavior. The third trigger was internal. At times Tanya was overcome with anxiety and depression at the loss of her mother. She desperately worried about her mother's safety and felt she needed to take care of her. The triggers caused an internal state of panic in Tanya, and her response was an immediate attempt to dampen her anxiety by the rhythmic motions of her genitals against objects. Tanya did not use her hands but humped anything she could find. With the help of her foster mother and hard work in therapy, she recognized that she was doing what she watched her mother do to men. This behavior did not lessen her panicky, sad or worried feelings, but transmit her to a dissociated state where she split off from her feelings and her body. In this dissociative state, she was oblivious to her environment and could no longer feel. With the help of her foster parents, Tanya was gradually able to identify the situations and feelings as they arose, and then engage in active strategies to diminish the feelings while staying present. Working with Tanya and the foster parents together, many activities were chosen and agreed upon that would be used when Tanya started feeling anxious and depressed. She learned to engage in fun and movement oriented activities with her foster parents, to leave the situation, or to talk about her thoughts and feelings with her foster parents and her therapist.

Additional factors that may encourage sexually-reactive behavior in children are: not getting clear messages about unacceptable sexual contact, and sexual abuse that is repressed as in the following vignette.

John's mother and father were drug addicts. He was removed from them when he was an infant, and lived with his paternal aunt and uncle. John's parents continued their drug use for the first six years of his life. While John was living with his aunt and uncle, his mother had sporadic visits with him, and his father disappeared. When he was around five years old, on one of these visits, he told his mother that his uncle's friend had made him suck on his penis, and this man had also sucked on John's penis two times. He said he liked the man very much and they had a really good time playing video games. The mother immediately told the Child Protective Service's worker. When the CPS worker asked John, he denied the story. The police also interviewed John to no avail.

John was put in therapy to see if this information would come forward. John's uncle and aunt selected the therapist and took John to the therapy appointments. The aunt and uncle insinuated to the therapist that the allegations were trumped up by the drug-addicted mother, who wanted to get the aunt and uncle in trouble. The therapist had no contact with the mother, and did not directly ask John at any time during the therapeutic process whether someone had engaged him in oral/genital contact. The therapist believed that if this had happened, the child himself would bring it up.

The aunt and uncle did not make the man who allegedly abused John leave the home. When John's mother would visit, she would ask him if the man who molested him was still at the house. John would tell the mother that he was, but then when the mother confronted the aunt and the uncle, John would generally retract his statements. On the occasions when he didn't retract his statements, the aunt and uncle would say they were not leaving the man alone with John. Worrying about her son's safety increased her strength to get off and stay off drugs. At the age of six and a half, John was able to return to his mother.

At the age of eight a compact disc was taken to the local police station near where the aunt and uncle lived with a note that the boy was John. On the CD, John was recognized as the victim of sodomy by an adult male and oral-genital contact by a woman. An investigation ensued. Neither the man or woman could be identified but it was determined that the man on the CD was not the same person who John had identified as molesting him when he was five. The pictures on the CD were of John at about three years old. Many of the pictures were in dark rooms with only a single light bulb. John often looked very drowsy or drugged.

As this information came out, and John was re-questioned about his earlier disclosure about molestation, he was very forthright about discussing the person who molested him. Now living separate from his aunt and uncle, he also acknowledged that the man stayed around his aunt and uncle's house, but said that he did not have any sexual contact with him again. John remembered three instances of oral/genial contact with the man. He said that the man was his very good friend and that he missed him. He said that the man was always very nice to him and didn't ever hurt him. He had no memories of not being forthright with Child Protective Service's and the Police. He remembered telling his mother about the oral-genital contact. John had no conscious memory of the sexual abuse portrayed on the CD.

While John's behavior had always been somewhat physically intrusive with all adults, the intrusive behavior became sexualized after the disclosure of the sexual abuse on the CD and discussion of the sexual abuse at his aunt and uncle's house. At times he would pounce on his mother and try to hump her as if simulating intercourse. He would also be all over her, trying to kiss her on the neck and face, and trying to touch her breasts. This would happen at home, in stores, and in the home of friends.

John entered therapy due to the sexual abuse on the CD, his lack of understanding that sexual contact by adults to children is abusive, and his uncontrolled sexual behavior with his mother. In assessing for dissociative phenomena, his mother was able to indicate that there were many times when John appeared to "space out." This was often under times of stress at home and at school, and also sometimes when he was playing. John's memory for recent and distant events was very spotty. His ability to handle conflict or heightened emotions was very poor. It would either send him into a rage, he would "space out," or he would want to go to sleep. He had very intense mood swings and could be physically overpowering to his mother at times of rage whereas generally he was a gentle child.

In working with John around the sexual behaviors, he indicated that he would get sexual feelings in his body and then would find himself jumping on his mother and humping her. It wasn't until she would yell at him to get off that he would become aware that he was on top of her. He said there was a gap in his memory between the sexual feelings and being on top of his mother. In thinking about his thoughts when he got the sexual feelings, he realized to his horror that he wanted to penetrate her anally. He said he knew it was not all right to want to be sexual with your mother but that the urges just swept over him. He said he didn't know where he got the thoughts and urges and did not want to have them.

John's use of dissociation to try to block the unacceptable thoughts and sexual urges for contact with his mother was quite receptive to behavioral interventions. After cataloging the sexually intrusive behaviors, the touching of his mother's breasts was selected as the target behavior to extinguish first. This was selected as it was the most frequent, happened in many locations, and was very distressing to his mother and others who observed it. After practice between John and his mother in the therapist's office, John was gently and consistently made aware by his mother when he was touching, or attempting to touch, her breasts, either with his hands, his face, his head, the top of his head, or his forehead. When this was brought to his attention, his mother would gently say "no," take hold of his hand and put it by his side. When John wanted to and it was appropriate, they played rock, paper, scissors in order to establish appropriate physical contact that was playful and enjoyable to both of them. After three weeks of work on this intrusive sexual behavior it ceased completely. Each time there was a court hearing that related in any way to the sexual abuse charges, there would be a re-emergence of the behavior, but to a lesser degree.

It is likely that the unconscious strivings were the result of sexual abuse by the man and woman shown on the CD and "his friend." John remained unable to remember anything about the

> abuse when he was three, perhaps due to it's unacceptable nature and/or that he was in a drugged state when it occurred and he therefore did not have access to it at a conscious level.

The above examples include children who were dissociative. However, it should be noted that most children with sexual behavior problems do not dissociate when engaging in the problematic sexual behaviors.

Children Who Engage in Extensive, Mutual Sexual Behaviors

Often distrustful, chronically hurt and abandoned by adults, children in this group relate best to other children. In the absence of close, supportive relationships with adults, they use their sexual behaviors to connect with other children. Children who engage in extensive, mutual sexual behaviors use sex as a way to cope with their feelings of abandonment, hurt, sadness, anxiety, and often despair. They do not coerce other children into sexual behaviors but find other similarly lonely children who will engage in sexual behaviors with them. Almost all of these children have been sexually and emotionally abused and neglected and look to other children to help meet their emotional needs and their need for physical contact.

Children in this group were previously sexually-reactive children. Children do not go from natural and healthy sexual behaviors to extensive, mutual sexual behaviors. First, they become confused and overwhelmed by the overt and covert sexuality to which they are exposed. Then, some come to use sex as a coping mechanism against their pain, despair, disillusionment, and lack of adult attachment figures (Johnson, 1988, 1999, 2000). The following vignette illustrates this coping mechanism.

> Raul was five and Maria was four when they were left in a room with a drunken older man. They were frequently left by their drug-addicted mother in motel rooms with people they didn't know. On this night it was late when they were left and Raul and Maria tried to go to bed on some blankets that they arranged on the floor. The drunken man in the bed was snoring very loudly. At one point during the night he woke up came toward them and yanked Maria up from the floor and put her into the bed with him. He pulled down her pants and tried to put his erect penis in her vagina. She screamed because it hurt and she didn't want him to do it. Raul got up and yelled at him and told him to stop. The man hit Raul

which caused him tumble to the side of the room where he hit his head. The man then let go of Maria, took another drink, and fell asleep. Raul and Maria tried to get out the door to leave, but couldn't. Unfortunately the man woke up again, and again tried to rape Maria. Raul was again unable to stop him, instead he yelled and then cried, begging him to not hurt his sister.

Clinging to each other for safety, the children went to sleep exhausted from the terror of the previous night. They were awakened by Child Protective Services and the police who interviewed them and removed them to foster care. From that time forward Raul and Maria engaged in simulating intercourse. As each foster parent found the children engaging in the sexual behavior they were placed in another home. At the fifth foster home treatment was sought.

They were brought to a treatment program for children who molested other children and their victims. After being in treatment for a short period of time, it became evident that Maria did not feel she was being molested, nor did Raul feel that he was molesting her. Maria said that she didn't want to tell people when she and Raul were engaging in sexual behavior with one another, because everybody got mad at Raul and punished him. She said, "It's not Raul's fault. I like to do it too." The children clearly felt safe when they were engaging in the sexual behavior, and did not see it as bad or wrong. Somehow, the desperate clinging to one another during the terror they felt in the motel room became their way of coping with their pain, sorrow and loneliness in foster care. They clung to each other when they felt most desperate and lost. There was no description by the children of sexual arousal or pleasure, only of emotional togetherness that gave them a sense that they were connected and therefore could survive.

As the therapists understood the fears of annihilation and desperation in the children and that the sexual behavior was a way of coping with these feelings, they helped them with alternative behaviors that attached them to their caregivers. When the children felt the emotional safety and physical security of loving, caring, containing and understanding adults, the sexual behavior dropped away. Each remained the others' closest and most trusted friend, but they were able to transfer their dependency needs onto trusted adults who cared for them. At six and seven years old there were no more concerns about Maria and Raul's sexual behavior.

Children Who Molest

The sexual behaviors of children in this category are frequent and pervasive. A growing pattern of sexual behavior problems is evident in their histories and intense sexual confusion is a hallmark of their thinking and behavior. Sexuality and aggression are closely linked in the thoughts and actions of these children. Unless the other child is too young to understand, children who molest use some type of coercion to get other children to participate in sexual behaviors. Bribery, trickery, manipulation, or emotional or physical coercion is generally used. Physical force is neither commonplace nor necessary as the children's victims are selected due to vulnerabilities, including developmental delays, social isolation, and emotional neediness. The victims may be older, younger, or the same age as the child who molests.

There is an impulsive and aggressive quality to many of the behaviors–including sexual behaviors–of children who molest. Generally, these children have problems in all areas of their lives. There is a progression for these children from healthy sexuality to sexually-reactive behaviors to molesting behaviors. Some of these children progress through all three groups prior to molesting (Johnson, 1988, 1999, 2000).

The following vignette concerning Eric provides a picture of a child who molests other children. His family background is replete with abuse and neglect, the modeling in his home gives a very distorted view of the place of sex in relationships, and emotional, physical and sexual violence is associated with all aspects of his family life.

> At nine years old Eric had forcibly penetrated the vagina of his five-year old sister with his penis on a minimum of three occasions. On the first occasion Eric's sister, Suzie, told her mother. Eric's mother beat him up and told him she'd kill him, if he did it again. Although his mother knew that Eric had great hostility towards his sister and had sexually abused his sister, she used Eric as a babysitter. It was on these occasions and others that Eric would physically terrify and sexually abuse his sister.
>
> Both children witnessed their father, Stan, beat up their mother and heard him raping her on many, many occasions. The children's father would repeatedly go into a drunken rage and emotionally and physically batter their mother accusing her of laziness, stupidity and infidelity. Eric was the scapegoat of both his mother and his father. His sister could do no wrong; Eric could do nothing right. His father physically and emotionally abused him from the

time he was very small. Both parents neglected Eric. Stan justified his behavior toward Eric in the same way he justified his violence towards his wife. He didn't like Eric's behavior or attitude and he was stupid and lazy.

Eric grew up fearing, hating, and desperately wanting his father to love him and his mother. He always felt confused about his mother. At times she would try to protect him from his father's wrath, and at other times she would stand by and say nothing while he was being beaten by his father. Eric learned not to trust anyone for emotional solace and physically safety.

Eric's mother, who was very dependent on Eric's father financially and emotionally, submitted to him sexually to keep the children from being homeless. Her anger at her husband became focused on Eric. When Eric entered the treatment program at nine, his mother could not even differentiate between Eric and his father. She would say, "He is just like his f__king father." While all of the negative projections from the father landed on Eric, Eric's mother could only see good in his sister. His sister was actually a very misbehaved and spoiled five-year old child "who got away with everything," thereby increasing the anger Eric felt toward her.

After Eric entered the treatment program it was determined that he had not been sexually abused, in any "hands on" way. But witnessing the physical aggression that often had sexual overtones, and hearing and feeling the sexual aggression toward his mother, Eric had paired the sex and anger that constantly surrounded him into a coping mechanism. When angry, confused, or when feeling emotionally hurt or abandoned, Eric used both physical and sexual aggression towards his sister to quell the feelings. His mother's strong projection onto him of being "just like his f__king father," was another strong catalyst for his hostile and sexually aggressive behavior as Eric played out the role assigned to him. While Eric was extremely angry at his mother for not protecting him, he was also angry at her for being victimized for so long by his father. While he was somewhat verbally and physically abusive to his mother, he took out the bulk of his anger and confusion at his mother and father on his sister. While many children who are angry at their parents might be emotionally and physically aggressive toward the favored sibling, Eric–with his father's model of hurting with sex–used sexual, emotional and physical methods to hurt his sister.

> With two years of clinical interventions with Eric and his mother and sister, they were able to live together in peace and harmony. There were no reported abusive sexual behaviors by Eric to his sister or anyone else.

The continuum of sexual behaviors as described above or elsewhere (Hall, Mathews, & Pearce, 1998; Pithers et al., 1998b) permits differentiation between children who molest and children with less serious sexual problems. This is essential in today's environment, as being mislabeled as a child who molests can mean:

- Removal from home
- Not being allowed to be alone with other children
- Not being allowed to attend regular classes in school
- Not being able to play freely in the neighborhood
- Being placed in therapy as an "offender"
- Not being allowed visits with the "victim" for an extended period of time
- Being put on a list of sex offenders

The term "sexual offender" is among the most highly charged labels in our culture. It can define a child's future employment and devastate his or her sexual development. Many children who are mislabeled also struggle to comprehend how their sexual behavior can fit the heinous crime of sexual offending (Chaffin & Bonner 1998). Megan's Law calls for the public notification of sex offenders (Freeman-Longo, 1996). States handle this notification process idiosyncratically (Freeman-Longo, 1996). By 1997, 19 states had mandated public notification of adjudicated juveniles who have sexually offended (Matson & Lieb, 1997). In Texas in 1999, there was a ten-year old on the list of registered sex offenders. His name and address were listed on the Internet (Johnson 2000).

CONCLUSIONS

There are a myriad of things that we still need to understand about the relationship between sexual abuse and children with sexual behavior problems. It is important to realize that not all children who molest have been sexually abused in a hands-on manner. Approximately one-half to two-thirds of children who molest were sexually victimized in a "hands-on" way. This should encourage the investigator or treatment provider to assess the children's environment more closely, not only focusing on hands-on sexual abuse by a sex offender. Not all children who are sexually abused will engage in any problematic sexual behaviors and only a very, very small number will molest other children when they are still children. As an overall strategy it is important to conceptualize children's sexual behavior along a continuum from natural and healthy to disturbed. Most children who do engage in problematic sexual behaviors are sexually-reactive. Children in the next largest group engage in extensive, but mutual sexual behaviors, and the smallest group is children who molest. It is important to determine which children may molest other children as the consequences are high–for both potential victims of abuse and for children who are inaccurately identified as potential molesters. In some states children can be listed on sex offender registries, and public notification is possible in some states. Careful assessment of problematic sexual behavior is essential to correctly identify and treat all children at risk and to identity the very small number who potentially may harm others.

REFERENCES

Bonner, B. (1998). Children with sexual behavior problems. Paper presented at the International Congress on Child Abuse and Neglect, Auckland, New Zealand.

Chaffin, M., & Bonner B. (1998). Don't shoot, we're your children: Have we gone too far in our response to adolescent sexual abusers and children with sexual behavior problems? *Child Maltreatment*, *4*(3), 314-316.

Conte, J., & Schuerman, J. (1987). The effects of sexual abuse on children: A multidimensional view. *Journal of Interpersonal Violence*, *2*, 380-390.

Finkelhor, D., Hotaling, G., Lewis, I.A., & Smith, C. (1990). Sexual abuse in a national survey of adult men and women: prevalence, characteristics, and risk factors. *Child Abuse & Neglect*, *14*, 19-28.

Freeman-Longo, R.E. (1996). Feel good legislation: Prevention or calamity? *Child Abuse & Neglect*, *20*, 95-101.

Freeman-Longo, R.E. (1996). Prevention or problem? *Sexual Abuse: A Journal of Research and Treatment*, *8*(2): 91-100.

Friedrich, W., & Chaffin, M. (2000). Developmental-systemic perspectives on children with sexual behavior problems. Paper presented at the Association for the Treatment of Sexual Abusers, San Diego.

Friedrich, W., Gramsch, P., & Damon, L. (1992). The Child Sexual Behavior Inventory: Normative and clinical comparisons. *Psychological Assessment*, *4*, 303-311.

Friedrich, W., & Luecke, W. (1988). Young school-age sexually aggressive children. *Professional Psychology Research and Practice*, *19*, 155-164.

Gray, A. (1996). Precursors to sexual aggression: Research implications for changing treatment of sexual misbehavior in young children. Paper presented at the Annual Conference of the Association for the Treatment of Sexual Abusers, Chicago, IL.

Gray, A., Busconi, A., Houchens, P., & Pithers, W.D. (1997). Children with sexual behavior problems and their caregivers: Demographics, functioning, and clinical patterns. *Sexual Abuse: A Journal of Research and Treatment*, *9*(4): 267-290.

Gray, A., Pithers, W.D., Busconi, A., & Houchens, P. (1999). Developmental and etiological characteristics of children with sexual behavior problems: Treatment implications. *Child Abuse & Neglect*, *23*, 601-621.

Hall, D.K., Mathews, F., & Pearce, J. (1998). Factors associated with sexual behavior problems in young children. *Child Abuse & Neglect*, *22*, 1045-1063.

Hanson, R.K., & Slater, S. (1988). Sexual victimization in the history of sexual abusers: A review. *Annals of Sex Research*, *1*, 485-499.

Johnson, T.C. (1988). Child perpetrators–children who molest other children: Preliminary findings. *Child Abuse & Neglect*, *12*, 219-229.

Johnson, T.C. (1988). The range of sexual behavior among children from natural and healthy to disturbed and sexually abusive children: Description of male and female children who molest. Paper presented at the 5th Annual Florida Child Abuse and Neglect Prevention Conference, St. Petersburg, FL.

Johnson, T.C. (1989). Female child perpetrators: children who molest other children. *Child Abuse & Neglect*, *13*, 571-585.

Johnson, T.C. (1998). *Child Sexual Behavior Checklist–Revised: Treatment exercises for abused children and children with sexual behavior problems*. South Pasadena CA: Author.

Johnson, T.C. (1998). Children who molest. In W.L Marshall, S.M. Hudson, Y.M. Fernandez, & T. Ward (Eds.), *Sourcebook of treatment programs for sexual offenders* (p. 344). New York: Plenum Press.

Johnson, T.C. (1998). *Understanding children's sexual behaviors–what's natural and healthy?* South Pasadena, CA: Author.

Johnson, T.C. (1999). *Understanding your child's sexual behavior*. Oakland, CA: New Harbinger Publications.

Johnson, T.C. (2000). Children with sexual behavior problems. *Sexuality Information and Education Council of the United States (SIECUS)*, *29*(1), 35-39.

Kaufman, J., & Zigler, E. (1987). Do abused children become abusive parents? *American Journal of Orthopsychiatry*, *57*(2), 186-192.

Kendall-Tackett, K.A., Williams, L.M., & Finkelhor, D. (1993). Impact of sexual abuse on children: A review and synthesis of recent empirical studies. *Psychological Bulletin*, *113*(1): 164-180.

Matson, S., & Lieb, R. (1997). Megan's law: A review of state and federal legislation. Olympia, WA: Washington State Institute for Public Policy.

Murphy, W.D., & Peters, J.M. (1992). Profiling Child Sexual Abusers: Psychological considerations. *Criminal Justice and Behavior*, *19*, 24-37.

Pithers, W.D., Gray, A., Busconi, A., & Houchens, P. (1998a). Caregivers of children with sexual behavior problems: Psychological and family functioning. *Child Abuse & Neglect*, *22*, 129-141.

Pithers, W.D., Gray, A., Busconi, A., & Houchens, P. (1998b). Children with sexual behavior problems: Identification of five distinct child types and related treatment considerations. *Child Maltreatment*, *3*(4), 384-406.

Hyposexuality and Hypersexuality Secondary to Childhood Trauma and Dissociation

Mark F. Schwartz, ScD
Lori Galperin, MSW, LCSW

SUMMARY. Childhood trauma can influence the bonding between the caretaker and the infant and thereby structure the stress response threshold. The capacity to utilize others as a form of self-soothing is determined by early attachments and also is critical to one's response to developmental stresses. The quality of early attachments strongly affects the capacity for adult intimacy. Early trauma and dissociative reactions have systematic effects on arousal, desire and pair-bonding, which are reviewed in this paper. A treatment model that addresses the early trauma and its aftereffects concerning intimacy and sexuality is discussed. *[Article copies available for a fee from The Haworth Document Delivery Service: 1-800-HAWORTH. E-mail address: <getinfo@haworthpressinc.com> Website: <http://www.HaworthPress.com> © 2002 by The Haworth Press, Inc. All rights reserved.]*

KEYWORDS. Sexual desire disorders, dissociation, attachment, trauma

---

Mark F. Schwartz and Lori Galperin are Clinical Directors, Masters and Johnson Clinic, St. Louis, MO.

Address correspondence to: Mark F. Schwartz, ScD, Masters and Johnson Clinic, 800 Holland Road, St. Louis, MO 63021 (E-mail: MFS96@aol.com).

[Haworth co-indexing entry note]: "Hyposexuality and Hypersexuality Secondary to Childhood Trauma and Dissociation." Schwartz, Mark F., and Lori Galperin. Co-published simultaneously in *Journal of Trauma & Dissociation* (The Haworth Medical Press, an imprint of The Haworth Press, Inc.) Vol. 3, No. 4, 2002, pp. 107-120; and: *Trauma and Sexuality: The Effects of Childhood Sexual, Physical, and Emotional Abuse on Sexuality Identity and Behavior* (ed: James A. Chu, and Elizabeth S. Bowman) The Haworth Medical Press, an imprint of The Haworth Press, Inc., 2002, pp. 107-120. Single or multiple copies of this article are available for a fee from The Haworth Document Delivery Service [1-800-HAWORTH, 9:00 a.m. - 5:00 p.m. (EST). E-mail address: getinfo@haworthpressinc.com].

CONCEPTUAL CONTEXT

Sexual desire is such a complex multi-factorial developmental system that there is little published on the subject that provides a sound conceptual base. Hyposexuality implies that the sexual response is consistently inhibited, typically accompanied by low initiatory behavior; while hypersexuality is the result of a low threshold for sexual responsiveness, often with obsessive-compulsive rituals of sexual expression that displace the unfolding of connection or caring for the partner. The rituals may also revolve around masturbation rather than partnered sex, or paraphilic sex, accompanied by a great deal of shame with a primary emphasis on relief of anxiety or tension. As with many addictive disorders, there can be a duality involving both over-control and out of control aspects that clinically seems to represent "two sides of the same coin," each with the common underlying organizing feature of fears of intimacy.

Often however, individuals are labeled or label themselves as hyposexual or hypersexual and the pattern becomes a dispositional trait or personality characteristic. Other characteristics may cluster around the central trait. Impulsiveness, rule breaking or passion may accompany hypersexuality, in contrast with rigidity, over control, distancing from others, and withdrawal into self for the inhibited individual with hyposexuality. In relationships, one individual can be labelled as hyposexual, and the deprived other appears to compulsively desire sex, with escalating polarization occurring until the labels become entrenched and indeed appear to represent antithetical extremes. Additionally, as a further pathway, certain co-morbid psychiatric illness, such as depression, clearly lowers sexual appetite and medications quite often amplify such effects, leading to further symptom exacerbation and self-labeling.

Sexual arousal and desire also define and are defined by the relational context. The experience of falling in love, for example, is often accompanied by hypersexuality, whereas relational boredom, fatigue, or hostility results in hyposexuality. Sexual behavior later in life is also potently influenced by antecedent childhood experiences that are related to pair-bonding. Fears of abandonment, engulfment, dependency, or being controlled, and deep feelings of self hatred all engender vulnerability in the capacity to form pair-bonds and subsequently, the capacity for sexual response.

Hyposexuality is most often used to describe individuals who do not have the desire for sex with a person they believe they love, such as a spouse or lover. Sexual desire is also quite responsive to situational performance failures, so for example, if the man repeatedly ejaculates rapidly, the woman may become hyposexual. In cases such as this, low sexual desire is easily reversed by performance successes or new partners.

Hypersexuality may frequently be dysfunctional. The hypersexual individual has been labeled by some writers as the "sex-addict" (Carnes, 1992), and the costs of such behavior can far outweigh the gratification. Yet such individuals seem compelled to continue, as with the high profile person who risks all in pursuit of sexual liaisons that are likely to ultimately be discovered. Typically, sexual acting out seems to produce an addictive "high," followed by shame. Some individuals' compulsive repertoires include illegal sexual activity with inappropriate partners, such as children or others who cannot give consent, or bizarre behavior such as inflicting pain or degradation on self or others. Compulsive sexual behavior can also include sex with objects; most notably more recently the pornography or cybersex addict may stay home masturbating, in preference to dating or spending time with a spouse. With compulsive hypersexuality, there seems to be a tolerance effect with an escalating level of intensity necessarily to get the same "hit," that seems to substantiate the characterization of "addiction." The individual becomes preoccupied with sexual behavior in an obsessional manner and establishes a compulsive habit to cope with escalating distress. Cognitive distortions further embed the behavior in the context of an increasingly self-destructive lifestyle.

ATTACHMENT DISORDER AND HYPOSEXUALITY AND HYPERSEXUALITY

Developmental psychopathology is a discipline that attempts to explore the developmental multi-determinants of adult psychiatric disorders by identifying those experiences that leave individuals vulnerable with respect to subsequent stressful life circumstances. The premise is that individuals establish varying vulnerabilities or resiliencies based on their first bonding experience. These early experiences then dictate the range of what individuals are reactive to, and to what degree they react. Some crucial determinants of the earliest bonding experience include the presence or absence of appropriate and timely response to the child's critical needs for attuned stimulation, soothing, attention, safety, affection, consistency, limit-setting, and touch. Bowlby's (1973) formulation was that attachment systems in infancy prepare the child to regulate arousal by effective utilization of others for self-soothing and self-control. In Alan Schore's (1994) words, development "essentially represents a number of sequentially mutually driven infant-caregiver processes which occur in a continuing dialectic between the maturing organism and the changing environment" (p. 64). This first relationship then acts as a "template" by which the individual enters into all subsequent emotional relationships. The result is varying levels of vulnerability and sensitivity to stressful events in which coping or "survival" strategies established during childhood become the root of either healthy functioning or adult psychopathology. For example, a child whose depressed mother is unresponsive to the child's smiles will disengage, become autonomically activated, and ultimately retreat into his own body for self-soothing (Tronick, 1989). This pattern becomes the basis of an adult intimacy disorder wherein the individual avoids using the pair-bond for comfort. This avoidance likewise translates into the sexual response realm. Unable to find soothing through intimacy, the individual remains unsatiated by orgasm.

Institutionalized children move through cycles of protest, despair and apathy, (Bowlby, 1980). Apathy may become characterological and is classically symptomatic of a long-term attachment disorder. Abused children will hypervigilently watch their mothers (Main, 1983), as if to take control by soothing their caregivers, but at the cost of relinquishing exploration of their environment and thereby establishing the capacity for mastery. These children are then more susceptible to cruelties from peers and neglect from teachers (Sroufe, 1989), which then further compounds their vulnerability to stresses. Chronically abused children may display classic signs of "Complex Post-Traumatic Stress Disorder" (Herman, 1992; van der Kolk, McFarland, & Weisaeth, 1996) that includes depression, anxiety, somatization, dissociation, addiction and relational/sexual difficulties with susceptibility to revictimization at different trajectory points in their development. In adult relationships, safety in close relationships is often maintained by anxiety-driven over-control, which typically causes relational power struggles.

One central component of Complex PTSD has been characterized by the term "disorders of the self" (Masterson & Klein, 1989), defined in part by the presence or absence of various self-functions. A self-function is a boundary defining capacity which arises from the individual's sense of self-perception, self-esteem, self-agency and self-efficacy, all of which effect the individual's appraisal of others' feedback and ultimately their overall interactions with others (Shane, Shane, & Gales,

1997). Given that sexual desire is an aspect of pair-bonding, factors contributing to or inhibiting the capacity for pair-bonding also define the parameters of sexual arousal. In a sense, sexual desire can be considered the self-function that is critical to how individuals define themselves in relation to others and how they bond with others.

When significant deficits and impairment of self function exist in a person, Greenspan (1996) suggests that such an individual "lacks critical capacities, called structural capacities which are central to self-regulation, (security, control, dependence), relating (affection, bonding, trust), pre-symbolic affective communicating (self in relation to others), representing and differentiating experiences and self observation (wishes and intentions) and boundary-defining gestures (mastery, social skills)" (pp. 57-59). Each of these structural capacities is central to sexual functioning. Initiating a pair-bond requires a realistic self-appraisal. If individuals consider themselves bad, defective, undeserving, damaged or unable to care for themselves, their ease in approaching potential mates would clearly be hampered. Boundary defining gestures, such as looking the other in the eye, social and dating skills are necessities in defining the nature of a dating interaction. After a contact is made, the individuals need to negotiate the boundaries of the relationship. An individual's need to care-take the other and ignore self-needs, to do things "perfectly" and seek the other's approval, are examples of manifestations of constraint or impairment in the arena of structural capacities. This type of formulation has led clinicians to conceptualize the entity of the sexual disorder more as a product of a courtship capacities deficit and consider the sexual problem as secondary to the proceptive love disorder (Money, 1986).

For individuals with impairment of self function, self-perceived ineptness in dating or mating interactions evokes feelings of incompetence, stupidity, dependence, self-hate, defectiveness and shame. It is as if the deeply ingrained affective patterns related to their first attachments activate feelings of defectiveness even when the current situation suggests the opposite. Such individuals are prone to self-sabotaging behavior as if to unconsciously recreate the early reflections of self received in primary relationships. Sexual desire in such cases can be largely anxiety driven, as the desire to conquer the other, or multiple others. In order to continually feel accepted, the individual is driven to compulsively seek affirmation of their acceptability as a way of combating deep self-hatred. Thus, hypersexual individuals starving for attention, affection, touch or validation, but without the structural capacities to substantially meet these needs, can achieve a tenuous, fleeting sense of reassurance and pseudo-intimacy. Hyposexuality, on the other hand, sets up a shield to protect the individual from anticipated rejection and prevent the vulnerability of allowing another close enough to recognize perceived self-defectiveness.

When the template formed was based on an early experience of terror related to abandonment or engulfment by the caretaker, potential relationships can activate intense survival fears. The individual experiences the contradictory emotions of sexual arousal while simultaneously feeling fear and a lack of deserving kindness and affection. The fears can then either shut down potential sexual arousal or potentiate it. It is therefore quite common for one individual to be both hypersexual and hyposexual within the same or different periods of their lives. Their extremes of responsiveness seem contradictory, but are actually a predictable adaptation to a set of complex overwhelming contradictory internal cognitive-affective, behavioral structures, evolved in response to original rejection, abandonment, neglect, assault, and resultant re-creations and misappraisals.

Treatment of such contradictory internal representations may require exposure to the original fearful childhood events (Foa & Kozak, 1986) that shaped such core self schema, with information reprocessing (Resnick & Schnicke, 1993) to permit realistic cognitions to replace the original fear-based ones (Fonagy et al., 1997). The model has been described as reliving-revising-revisiting (Glaser, personal correspondence; Schwartz & Gay, 1996), in that clients reexperience the fears and other overwhelming affect in the safety and containment of the therapist's office. They are then coached to question their original conclusions about self, sometimes utilizing hypnosis, internal family systems therapy (Schwartz, 1995), eye-movement desensitization and reprocessing (EMDR; Shapiro, 1995), psycho-dramatic or gestalt therapies. In the revisiting stage they are taught self-functions and repair of structural capacities that are deficient from developmental deprivation and misappraisals.

Also highly critical to sexual arousal is the capacity for affect regulation that is initially established by the external responsiveness and guidance of caregivers. When the caregiver is attuned to the excitatory and inhibitory cycles of the child, an internalized sense of control is established. In neglectful or abusive families, affect regulation is often inconsistent, over-controlled or non-existent. A lack of such internal control can underlie the over control and/or out of control of sexual impulsiveness.

As a child matures, parents lend their capacities to apprise self-functions to the child, providing mirroring. This capacity is described by

Fonagy et al. (1997) as "reflective function." Relative to sexual unfolding, if, for example, a child's touching of her own genitals is witnessed by a parent and responded to with a punitive affective response, the child comes to encode sexual urges as bad. If, as another variation, a child's father is caught in an affair by the mother and the child views the mother having a violent response, the sexuality of men generically can become negatively coded. Even though the context of these events can be lost to memory, the affect can be stored in the unconscious representational systems related to future pair-bonding of the child.

Prolonged negative affects, affective dyscontrol by caregivers, and habitual caregiver hostility often lead to fear of the caregiver. The need for safety and bonding is then contradicted by fear, both very strong primary emotions. The result is often psychopathology and resultant intimacy disorder. Children for whom this is the case display failed attachment and lack the capacity to understand the minds and feelings of others (Fonagy et al. 1997). In extreme cases, such a severe mixture of primary emotions can result in paraphilia; the individual is not aroused by other adults but alternative stimuli, e.g., children, shoes, or particular objects. It is as if sexuality emerges within a context of shame, fear and self-hatred and thereby becomes "hardwired" to deviant substitute objects during puberty. At the other extreme, reflective function that associates negative emotions with emerging sexuality results in too much inhibition, stigmatization or isolation from social interaction, and suppression of affect. In such cases, anxiety can become amplified and result in avoidance and/or inhibition of natural bodily functions. When, however, individuals feel a build up of tension from unresolved feelings of rage, anxiety, helplessness, self-loathing and/or emptiness, they will then turn to sexual behavior as a temporary distraction to provide interruption of the dysphoric state, resulting in restoration of control and a temporary feeling of relief from the emptiness, or self-soothing. A sense of calm and relief ensues, perpetuating the over-control/out of control cycle.

SEXUAL TRAUMA AND DISSOCIATION AND SEXUAL AROUSAL

Sexual abuse is a particularly pernicious form of trauma in that it disrupts the development of the self-system, affect regulation and a sense of safety in interpersonal relationships at critical stages in development. When sexual abuse occurs, sexual arousal often becomes activated prematurely, but within a context of betrayal, fear, confusion, shame, and violence. The oft accompanying destruction of the sense of safety within the child's home, body and of trust in the caretaker's ability to provide protection, and trust in significant adult figures generally, creates enduring feelings of personal vulnerability. Self-perception is damaged, and a sense of badness or core defectiveness results (Summit, 1983) alongside a sense of powerlessness and loss of control over body as well as environment. These losses and the associated fears and anxieties that accompany them interfere with the developing capacity for intimacy.

The long-term effects of early abuse on adult sexuality vary. They depend on the child's age, duration of the abuse, relationship with the perpetrator, sex of victim and victimizer, previous trauma, and the way the event is processed, as well as the counteracting effects of positive, reinforcing early attachments and the stability of the family environment. The most common response is hyposexuality in close intimate relationships and hypersexuality with new partners. The latter is often a reenactment of the original incident repeated over and over. Stoller (1975) has characterized this element of compulsive reenactment as "perversion," and describes how it provides a sense, though perhaps misplaced, of "triumph over tragedy," in the sense that, seemingly, this time the victim chooses, rather than submits. The drivenness of the need to repetitively reenact a once traumatic event can hardly be said to signify resolution. Instead, it is as if the brain is unable to assimilate the overwhelming, confusing and often contradictory behavior, affect, sensations, and knowledge implicit in the sexual abuse and thereby drives the person to repeat in order to finally establish a solution. While frenzied reenactment constitutes phase one, once the individual becomes intimate, trauma-engendered core fears of closeness and hatred of self become activated, neutralizing sexual desire. Thus, hypersexuality gives way to hyposexuality.

Braun's (1985) BASK model of dissociation, that is, the segmentation of behavior, affect, sensation, and knowledge is extremely applicable to sexual arousal. Dissociation of affect might include experiencing feelings of terror, numbness or confusion without any apparent cause, or experiencing affect incongruent with the present situation. It has been noted that many men in this culture highly dissociate from affect. Unaware of a myriad of emotions and feeling distant and disconnected from their partners, sex is experienced as a need for ejaculation rather than intimacy. Some individuals can have sex without affection because of dissociated affect. On the other hand, a person might experience sexual apathy or impotence because the individual is terrified but unaware of it. Unable to use fear or terror as a signal, some individuals attempt to "perform," but genital vasocongestion is blocked by fear.

Dissociation secondary to childhood trauma also becomes a mediator of sexual desire. Behavioral dissociation is, for example, common with men who perform anonymous sex with strangers whom they often do not like nor find attractive, men who put their penises through holes, without knowing who is on the other side, for the purpose of oral genital contact, or women who function repeatedly as prostitutes. In some instances, such dissociated behavior serves as a reenactment of the original trauma. A part of the self will revisit the experience of childhood rape repetitively, to repeat the danger and excitement, in an attempt to complete the stress response cycle.

Dissociation of sensation may manifest in numbness, headaches or sickness or pelvic pain with no medical explanation. Touching one's partner sexually may be experienced as comparable to touching an inanimate object by one person, while to another, it may signal a need to immediately orgasm. The sensory systems of sexually traumatized individuals are particularly prone to injury. When sexual unfolding occurs prematurely and within a context of force, coercion, brutality and objectification, elements become intertwined that under healthy, developmentally appropriate circumstances would not be linked. This phenomenon, in its myriad manifestations, is known as trauma bonding (Schwartz, Galperin, & Masters, 1993). The most damaging fusion of elements perhaps, is the pairing of terror with sexual arousal. One client with dissociative identity disorder described how she experiences this phenomenon relative to the responses of her internal self system:

> I don't know that we've ever experienced true sexual arousal–only fear arousal, arousal driven by terror, anxiety or excitement that is basically over-stimulation. When we feel these, it translates into a physical response in the vaginal area.

For this client, natural unfolding of sexual response at a normal developmental level was brutally preempted by the repeated, unpredictable evoking of sexual responsiveness by others who exercised virtual life and death control over her. When the arousal potential of the child is prematurely forced to unfold at the behest of an all powerful adult using that child's body as a receptacle for hostilely driven release, arousal is equated with danger. The weight of an adult body crushing a child, a silencing hand over nose and mouth, and a whispered threat not to tell, or else . . . is hardly the stuff of romance, or is it? So much of what passes for "erotica" recapitulates themes of subjugation, infliction of pain and disconnection. One wonders whether the target market is not chosen with a clear sense of capitalistic pandering to the drivenness that accompanies sexual pursuits by individuals who recapitulate the insults or injuries to their unfolding affectional and/or sexual system during their early development. Whenever child sexual abuse occurs at the hands of trusted others upon whom the child has previously relied for safety, the degree of dissociation and self fragmentation required to contend with it is exponentially increased, especially where the child must continue to rely upon these others. Compounding the original damage, later in life, the individuals may view their trauma bonded sexual responses as "evidence" that original perpetrators were correct in their ascribing of "innate badness" to them, as part of the ostensible rationale for the original abuse.

Van der Kolk and van der Hart (1989) have suggested that dissociation can be primary, secondary, or tertiary. In the arena of sexual abuse, primary dissociation results in persons feeling objectified and depersonalized and, in turn, considering others as objects to use for their narcissistic satisfaction. They "fuck" or are "fucked," to use the colloquial term, but typically feel the pleasure of physical release with minimal bonding or connectedness with the partner, and also with less satiety. Primary dissociation is exemplified by some ambisexual individuals (Masters & Johnson, 1970) who will have sex with men or women without any specific preference, attraction or bonding. The individual appears numb and disconnected from self and others, using orgasm as an escape from emptiness. In some such individuals' histories, they survived overwhelming experiences by dissociation, and now appear to dissociate involuntarily. Many individuals seem to have less extreme, unconscious fears of the vulnerability of being close and nude with lovers, and dissociate. In order to then feel, they require illicitness, pain, novelty or romance to experience arousal.

Secondary dissociation results in a person having the sense of leaving their body and not actually being present for sexual interchange because of the terror of being close or due to flashbacks to prior abuse. The individual either experiences hyposexuality and is numb, or "bypasses" the emotions and is able to perform with many partners in a mechanical way, with seemingly little desire or arousal. Typically, this was the defense utilized when no escape was possible from prior physical onslaught and now, even chosen opportunities with select partners still contain triggers–certain touch, words, tastes, smells, sensations–that automatically cue the protective response of dissociation.

Finally, tertiary dissociation implies fragmentation of the self into disparate ego states (Watkins and Watkins, 1971) that function at cross purposes. When there is a history of sexual abuse, often there is a part of self described as a "seducer or seductress," which will "conquer" desired partners utilizing sex. However, after the partner is committed, the body is often hyposexual. Ironically, but not unpredictably, once genuine intimacy and trust enter the picture, it may be more difficult to override fear through reliance on more robotic parts of self. Other aspects of tertiary dissociation result when encapsulated child parts that are frozen in time "come out" during sex with cognitions and affect that are trauma coded, e.g., "sex is yucky or dirty." Obviously, in such cases, some measure of trauma resolution and integration of split off parts of self is essential before attempting sexual therapies.

When there is secure attachment and minimal childhood trauma, an individual develops pride in their self-identity, their gender, and their sexuality. They are able to move into an intimate relationship, use others for self-soothing, and internalize self-soothing and other capacities, thereby evolving both autonomy and interpersonal relatedness. They continue to know more of their identity through close relationships and do not fear losing themselves in their dependencies, nor their partners in their solitude. In such cases, sexuality becomes a natural manifestation of affection, with fluidity in appetite, resembling that for food.

Conversely, damage to the self-system results in activation of fears of intimacy when the individual is in a position to be sexually vulnerable. Individuals described as having avoidant attachment by Ainsworth and her colleagues (1978) seem to develop a long-term characterological avoidance of closeness. Bowlby (1980) notes that "when such an individual attempts to live his life without the love and support of others, he tries to become emotionally self-sufficient and may be diagnosed as narcissistic or having a false self," as described by Winnicott (1949/1975). Such narcissism was exemplified by a recent client who had multiple affairs with his customers in his office while his wife was pregnant. He stated, "I am not sure I love my wife or that I have ever loved or am capable of loving." Instead, he was hypersexual and seduced women compulsively, as if sustaining a cohesive sense of self was dependent on their presumed receptivity. When his mother came in for a family assessment, she displayed active avoidance of her grandchild. When we inquired about this behavior, she acknowledged that after her husband left her with the young children as the result of an affair with another woman, she never again "allowed herself to love anyone or anything." When this same client entered marital therapy with his wife, we noted that he was consistently hyposexual.

We propose that the treatment of a specific triad of symptoms–disorders of self, affect regulation, and interpersonal relationships–requires highly individualized trauma-based and integrative therapies. Such treatment should focus on the resolution and integration of developmentally overwhelming events in a time-limited format. A strong relationship with the therapist is requisite for such work. Directive techniques for neutralizing therapy, life and relationship interfering behavior (Linehan, 1993) can be utilized to counter common resistances. This phase of treatment is followed by placing the individual into therapy with the partner or spouse and using the relationship as a further vehicle for change (Schwartz & Masters, 1988). The couple is given specific suggestions by a co-therapy team to catalyze increasing levels of intimacy in and out of the bedroom. The roadblocks, structural deficits or fears that have interfered with sexual desire usually manifest themselves, and directive psychotherapy is used to intervene and teach new skills. Cognitive behavioral therapies are utilized to enhance the couple's skills at intimate interchange such as: problem-solving, demonstrativeness, responsiveness to other's needs, creativity in socializing, methods of dealing with long-term hostility and ambivalences with closeness, vulnerability, trust and bonding. Each therapy session is both diagnostic and therapeutic, because more information about the individual's structural deficits and how they become manifest in the relationship is gleaned from processing the events and interchanges of the prior day. The therapist actively (1) confronts the destructive transaction, (2) points out it's origin, and (3) puts in current perspective it's potentially destructive consequences, (4) offers skills to improve or change the behavior, and (5) provides suggestions of ways of practicing the new skills between the sessions. When the client becomes stuck or unable to benefit from cognitive-behavioral suggestions, the stuck point is used as a window into deeper unconscious conflicts, not completely resolved from the individual therapy. At this juncture, trauma-based exposure and information reprocessing therapies are used with the spouse in the room and the couple is sent home with suggestions of how to further share emotions and responses emerging from the deeper work. In this way, intimacy is facilitated in the therapist's office–*in vivo*–and its building is continued between sessions. Suggestions for sexual intimacy through sensate focus exercises (Masters & Johnson, 1970) are integrated into the newly created safety and closeness of the intimate relationship, reversing many of the sensory integration issues that began in early attachment deficits or childhood trauma. Such exercises also emphasize shifting attention to the partner using mindfulness, which typically begins to neutralize the automatic dissociative patterns, and allows for novel and ameliorative experience in the here and now.

REFERENCES

Ainsworth, M., Biehas, M., Wateres, E., & Wall, S. (1978). *Patterns of attachment.* Hillsdale, NY: Erlbaum.

Bowlby, J. (1973). *Separation: Anxiety and anger. Attachment and loss, vol. 2.* New York: Basic Books.

Bowlby, J. (1980). *Loss: Sadness and depression. Attachment and loss, vol. 3.* New York: Basic Books.

Braun, B.G. (1985). The transgenerational incidence of dissociation and multiple personality disorder, A preliminary report. In R.P. Kluft (Ed.), *Childhood antecedents of multiple personality,* (pp. 127-150). Washington, DC: American Psychiatric Press.

Carnes, P. (1992). *Out of the shadows: Understand sexual addiction.* Centre City, MN: Hazelden Educational Materials.

Foa, E. B., & Kozak, M. (1986). Emotional processes of fear: Exposure to corrective information. *Psychological Bulletin, 99,* 20-35.

Fonagy, P., Target, M., Steele, M., Steele, H., Leigh, T., Levinson, A., & Kennedy, R. (1997). Morality, disruptive behavior, borderline personality disorder, crime and their relationship to security of attachment. In L. Atkinson & K. J. Zucker (Eds.), *Attachment and psychopathology* (pp. 223-274). New York: Guilford Press.

Greenspan, S. (1996). *Developmentally based psychotherapy.* Madison, CT: International University Press.

Herman, J.L. (1992). *Trauma and recovery.* New York: Basic Books.

Herman, J.L., Perry, J.C, & van der Kolk, B.A. (1989). Childhood trauma in borderline personality disorder. *American Journal of Psychiatry, 146,* 490-495.

Linehan, M. (1993). *Cognitive-behavioral therapy for borderline personality disorder.* New York: Guilford Press.

Main, M. (1983). Exploration, play, and cognitive functioning related to infant-mother attachment. *Infant Behavior & Development, 6,* 167-174.

Masters, W.H., & Johnson, V. (1970). *Human sexual inadequacy.* Boston: Little Brown.

Masterson, J., & Klein, R. (Eds.) (1989). *Psychotherapy of the disorders of self.* New York: Brunner/Mazel.

Money, J. (1986). *Lovemaps: Clinical concepts of sexual erotic health and pathology, paraphilia, and gender transposition of childhood, adolescence, and maturity.* New York: Irvington.

Resnick, P.A., & Schnicke, M.K. (1993). *Cognitive processing therapy for rape victims.* Newbury Park, CA: Sage Publications.

Schwartz, C.R. (1995). *Internal family systems therapy.* The Guilford Press.

Schwartz, M.F., Galperin, L., & Masters, W.H. (1995). Sexual trauma within the context of traumatic and inescapable stress and poisonous pedagogy. In M. Hunter (Ed.), *The sexually abused male, vol. 3* (pp. 1-17). Thousand Oaks, CA: Sage Publications.

Schwartz, M.F., & Gay, P. (1996). Physical and sexual abuse, neglect and early disorder symptoms. In M.F. Schwartz & L. Cohn (Eds.), *Sexual abuse and eating disorders* (pp. 91-108). New York: Brunner/Mazel.

Schwartz, M.F., & Masters, W.H. (1988). Inhibited sexual desire: The Masters & Johnson Institute treatment model. In S. Leiblum, & R. Rosen, (Eds.), *Sexual desire disorders* (p. 229-242). New York: Guilford Press.

Shane, M., Shane, E., & Gales, M. (1997). *Intimate attachments: Toward a new self psychology.* New York: Guilford Press.

Shapiro, F. (1995). *Eye movement desensitization and reprocessing: Basic principles, protocols, and procedures.* New York: Guilford Press.

Schore, A. (1994). *Affect regulation and the origin of self.* Hillsdale, NY: Erlbaum.

Stoller, R. (1975). *Perversion: The erotic form of hatred.* New York: Pantheon.

Sroufe, L.A. (1989). Infant-caregiver attachment and patterns of adaptation in preschool: The roots of maladaptation and competence. In M. Perlmutter (Ed.), *Minnesota symposium in child psychology, vol. 16* (pp. 41-83). Hillsdale, NJ: Lawrence Erlbaum Associates.

Summit, R.C. (1983). The child sexual abuse accommodation syndrome. *Child Abuse and Neglect, 7,* 177-193.

Tronick, E. (1989). Emotions and emotional communication in infants. *American Psychologist, 44,* 112-119.

Van der Kolk, B., McFarland, A.C., & Weisaeth, L. (Eds.) (1996). *Traumatic stress: The effects of overwhelming experience on the mind, body & society.* New York: Guilford Press.

Van der Kolk, B.A., & van der Hart, O. (1989). Pierre Janet and the breakdown of adaptation in psychological trauma. *American Journal of Psychiatry, 146,* 1530-1540.

Watkin, J.G. (1971). The affect bridge: A hypnoanalytic technique. *International Journal of Clinical Hypnosis, 19,* 21-27.

Winnicott, D.W. (1949/1975). Mind and its relation to the psycho-soma. In D.W. Winnicott, *Through pediatrics to psychoanalysis* (pp. 243-254). New York: Basic Books.

Traumatic Experiences: Harbinger of Risk Behavior Among HIV-Positive Adults

Cheryl Gore-Felton, PhD
Cheryl Koopman, PhD

SUMMARY. Far more than in the general population, people living with HIV tend to report experiencing traumatic life events, particularly those that are violent and abusive. The majority of AIDS cases in the United States and globally result from either unprotected sexual intercourse or the use of contaminated injection drug needles. This study examined the relationship between trauma history, trauma-related symptoms, and sexual risk behavior. The sample included 64 men and women living

Cheryl Gore-Felton is affiliated with the Department of Psychiatry & Behavioral Medicine, Medical College of Wisconsin, Milwaukee, WI.

Cheryl Koopman is affiliated with the Department of Psychiatry & Behavioral Sciences, Stanford University, School of Medicine, Stanford, CA.

Address correspondence to: Cheryl Gore-Felton, PhD, Medical College of Wisconsin, Center for AIDS Intervention Research (CAIR), 2071 North Summit Avenue, Milwaukee, WI 53202 (E-mail: cgore@mcw.edu).

The authors appreciate the contributions of Luther Brock, Xin-Hua Chen, Margaret Chesney, Catherine Classen, Sue Dimiceli, Michael Edell, Michele Gill, Peea Kim, David Lewis, and Jose Maldonado and the men and women who served as participants in this research.

This research was supported by NIMH Minority Postdoctoral Fellowship Award R1MH54930A, R01 MH54930 (principal investigator, David Spiegel, MD), and Center Grant P30 MH52776 (principal investigator, Jeffrey A. Kelly, PhD).

[Haworth co-indexing entry note]: "Traumatic Experiences: Harbinger of Risk Behavior Among HIV-Positive Adults." Gore-Felton, Cheryl, and Cheryl Koopman. Co-published simultaneously in *Journal of Trauma & Dissociation* (The Haworth Medical Press, an imprint of The Haworth Press, Inc.) Vol. 3, No. 4, 2002, pp. 121-135; and: *Trauma and Sexuality: The Effects of Childhood Sexual, Physical, and Emotional Abuse on Sexuality Identity and Behavior* (ed: James A. Chu, and Elizabeth S. Bowman) The Haworth Medical Press, an imprint of The Haworth Press, Inc., 2002, pp. 121-135. Single or multiple copies of this article are available for a fee from The Haworth Document Delivery Service [1-800-HAWORTH, 9:00 a.m. - 5:00 p.m. (EST). E-mail address: getinfo@haworthpressinc.com].

with HIV/AIDS. An examination of trauma symptoms and sexual risk behavior indicated that moderate to severe trauma symptoms were significantly correlated with unprotected sexual intercourse during the past three months. Moreover, reliving the traumatic event (i.e., experiencing flashbacks, having nightmares) was significantly and positively associated with having more partners in the past 3 months. Greater symptoms of intrusion and avoidance were associated with unprotected sex. After controlling for demographic factors, multiple regression analysis indicated that greater severity of sexual coercion, greater intrusion symptoms, and less avoidant symptoms were positively associated with greater sexual risk behavior. Thus, reducing trauma symptoms among adults with moderate to severe symptoms may be a particularly effective HIV-prevention intervention for adults living with HIV/AIDS.

KEYWORDS. HIV, trauma, risk behavior, stress

At the end of 1999, there were an estimated 33.6 million people living with HIV or AIDS. Worldwide surveillance data indicate that AIDS has been diagnosed in virtually every country, and HIV infection and illness have increased at alarming rates in developing countries in sub-Saharan Africa and Asia (Joint United Nations Programme on HIV/AIDS World Health Organization, 1998). In the United States, the estimated number of deaths among persons with HIV decreased by 25% during 1995-1996 (Centers for Disease Control and Prevention [CDC], 1996), by 46.4% in 1997 (Holmes, 1998), and by 21% from 1997-1998 (Martin, Smith, Mathews, & Ventura, 1999).

Although the number of new HIV infections has declined (CDC, 1999; Holmes, 1998; Martin et al., 1999), ethnic minority groups in the United States represent a disproportionately high percentage of people with AIDS. African-Americans represent 12.2% of the total population (U.S. Census Bureau, 1999), however, they constitute nearly 37% of the AIDS cases reported through June 1999 (CDC, 1999). Similarly, people who are Hispanic/Latino compose 11.6% of the total population (U.S. Census Bureau, 1999), but represent over 18% of the AIDS cases (CDC, 1999). From July 1998-June 1999, African-American adults and children represented 46% of the new AIDS cases (CDC, 1999). Hispanic/Latino adults and children represented over 19% of the new AIDS cases (CDC, 1999).

The majority of AIDS cases in the United States and globally results from either unprotected sexual intercourse or the use of contaminated injection drug needles. Both means of transmission can be prevented through behavioral change. Since HIV transmission requires exposure to an HIV-positive person, prevention efforts need to target HIV-positive populations. Thus, understanding factors associated with risk among HIV-positive individuals will be key to developing effective prevention interventions.

Far more than in the general population, people living with HIV tend to report experiencing traumatic life events, particularly those that are violent and abusive. Indeed, in a nationally representative probability sample of 2,864 HIV-positive adults being physically harmed by a partner or other person close to them was reported by 21 percent of the women and 12 percent of men who have sex with men (Zierler et al., 2000). Moreover, there is evidence suggesting that experiences of physical assault, rape and robbery are more prevalent among seropositive inner-city African American women compared to their uninfected counterparts (Kimerling et al., 1999). In a study conducted in California, 61% of the men and women living with HIV reported a traumatic experience severe enough to meet the PTSD definition for a stressful event (Gore-Felton, Butler, & Koopman, 2001). Indeed, in a study among HIV-positive and negative women, significantly more HIV-positive women (79%) reported experiencing violence compared to 21% of the women who were HIV-negative (Axelrod, Myers, Durvasula, Wyatt, & Cheng, 1999). Men who have sex with men are also vulnerable to violence, particularly domestic violence. Such men who are HIV-positive and in abusive relationships often find it difficult to leave the relationships or engage in safer behavior (Letellier, 1996).

Among female sex partners of male drug users, a substantial proportion reported histories of rape, assault, and threat of assault. These traumatic events were associated with HIV risk such that women who had been raped or threatened with assault were more likely to have multiple sex partners and engage in unprotected anal sex (He, McCoy, Stevens, & Stark, 1998). Indeed, some researchers are asserting that violence assessment, particularly domestic violence, is an important adjunct for effective HIV prevention (Klein & Birkhead, 2000). The association between trauma and HIV was also found among 52 HIV-symptomatic patients when 65% reported histories of childhood sexual/physical abuse (Allers & Benjack, 1991). Furthermore, the characteristic abuse symptoms of chronic depression, sexual compulsivity, revictimization, and substance abuse have been identified as barriers to HIV education and intervention for survivors (Allers, Benjack, White, & Rousey, 1993). In a sample of 425 young men who had sex with men, a lifetime history of forced sex was significantly associated with the likelihood of having unsafe anal sex in the six months prior to the interview (Lemp et al., 1994). Similarly, in a study examining high risk sexual behavior among 182 men of Puerto Rican ancestry living in New York City who had sex with men, men with a history of childhood sexual abuse were significantly more likely to engage in receptive anal sex and to do so without protection (Carballo-Diéguez & Dolezal, 1995). This is consistent with research indicating that men with a childhood sexual abuse (CSA) history were more likely to engage in unprotected receptive anal intercourse, trade sex for money, drugs, or place to stay, report being HIV positive, and report being hit by a relationship partner (Gore-Felton, Brondino, Benotsch, Kalichman, & Cage, in submission). In addition, in a study of men who have sex with men, men with a CSA history were more likely to report sexually coercive events involving unprotected anal intercourse (Kalichman et al., 2001), which is the highest sexual risk behavior for HIV transmission.

Post-traumatic stress symptoms complicate not only responses to traumatic stressors themselves, but also co-morbid medical and psychiatric problems, including HIV infection. The prevalence of posttraumatic stress disorder (PTSD) in the general population is about 9% (Breslau, Davis, Andreski, & Peterson, 1991); partial PTSD is estimated to be close to 30% (Weiss et al., 1992). The rates are likely to be higher among those with HIV infection, due in part to the lifestyle associated with elevated disease risk. Indeed, among African-American HIV-positive women, 62% reported experiencing at least one traumatic life event with 35% of the sample meeting the full criteria for PTSD diagnosis (Kimerling et al., 1999). Moreover, 87.9% reported symptoms of re-experiencing the traumatic event, 73.5% reported avoidance and 70.4% reported symptoms of hyperarousal. One hypothesis is that the psychological symptoms (e.g., intrusion, hyperarousal, and avoidance) associated with a traumatic experience may interfere with the individual's ability to integrate safer patterns of interpersonal and personal functioning.

It is important to understand the link between trauma and substance use because substance use and sexual risk behaviors are the principal routes for transmission of HIV infection (Des Jarlais & Friedman, 1998; Hearst & Hulley, 1988) and they tend to co-occur. It is argued that alcohol and other drugs have a direct causal effect on sexual behavior and condom use by impairing one's judgment about possible risks, disinhibiting oneself physically and psychologically, and making one less sensitive to the concerns of a partner (Strunin & Hingson, 1992). High-risk sexual behavior is strongly related to substance use (Kalichman, 2000). Thus, use of drugs and alcohol can increase the risk of becoming HIV-infected when the sexual partner has HIV infection (Ostrow et al., 1990; Penkower et al., 1991). Indeed, the majority of persons with AIDS have reported one or more sexual/IV drug use risk behavior as a likely route of transmission of HIV (CDC, 1994), and risk behaviors continue among some persons already HIV-infected. Even among well-educated employed women who are not intravenous drug users, 60% engaged in unprotected sexual activity after learning that they were HIV positive (Brown & Rundell, 1990). Importantly, many men who have sex with men and persons using intravenous drugs have changed their risk behaviors in response to the threat of AIDS (Catañia et al., 1992; Des Jarlais & Friedman, 1988). However, even after reducing high-risk sex and drug use behaviors, relapse often occurs (Des Jarlais, Friedman, & Casriel, 1990; Stall, Ekstrand, Pollack, McKusick, & Coates, 1990). One explanation may be that trauma-related stress was not assessed and therefore, symptoms of stress were not addressed in the intervention. It should be noted that the comorbidity of PTSD and substance abuse is high (Keane & Wolfe, 1990; Kulka et al., 1990). Indeed, 59% of women with trauma histories attending a drug rehabilitation clinic experienced symptoms that met criteria for PTSD (Fullilove et al., 1993).

Better understanding of the association between trauma and HIV risk behavior will assist in the development of successful interventions that facilitate HIV risk behavior by addressing underlying issues related to traumatic experiences. As the medical management of people living with HIV and AIDS continues to improve, more and more HIV-positive people are living healthier, longer lives, which increases the threat of secondary infections. Indeed, there is evidence suggesting that HIV-positive men and women who experienced childhood sexual trauma engage in behaviors that put themselves and others at increased risk for HIV transmission. Although researchers have theorized that trauma symptoms associated with the childhood traumatic event lead to risky behavior, the only data linking trauma symptoms to risk behavior has been obtained on men (Carballo-Diéguez & Dolezal, 1995; Gore-Felton et al., in submission; Kalichman et al., 2001; Lemp et al., 1994). Moreover, there has been no research reported to date examining the impact of trauma other than childhood sexual abuse on HIV-risk behavior. This is an important omission for two reasons. First, traumatized HIV-positive populations appear to be at increased risk for HIV transmission. Second, there is no effective HIV-risk reduction intervention designed to address the trauma-related issues, which may put one at increased risk. Consequently, understanding the association between traumatic experiences, trauma symptoms, and risk behavior will assist researchers and health service providers in developing effective HIV prevention interventions. Therefore, this study will examine trauma symptoms, substance use, and the types of trauma experiences associated risk behavior among an ethnically diverse and gender-balanced sample of HIV-positive men and women. To our knowledge, there has not been a study examining the relationship between trauma and sexual risk behavior among a diverse sample of HIV-positive adults.

METHODS

Participants

This study was part of an ongoing randomized clinical trial designed to examine the effect of group psychotherapy on quality of life and health behavior among adults living with HIV/AIDS. All participants completed informed consent forms prior to completing study questionnaires. This study examined the baseline questionnaires, prior to randomization, of 64 participants who completed self-report measures on demographics, trauma history, trauma symptoms, substance use, and sexual behavior. The sample was recruited through newspaper advertisements and medical clinics. The sample was ethnically diverse such that 49% identified themselves as Caucasian, 33% as African-American, 7% as Latino, and 11% as other. Sixty-one percent (61%) of the sample was female (N = 39); the average age was 38.7 years; 20% of the sample did not graduate from high school; 87% had household incomes less than $20,000 year; 28% were diagnosed with AIDS; and 57% identified as heterosexual.

Measures

All participants completed a demographic/medical questionnaire that assessed variables such as age, income, gender, and ethnicity. Medical information regarding confirmation of HIV status was verified by written documentation from physicians. Those participants with CD4+ lymphocyte count below 200 were considered to meet criteria for AIDS (CDC, 1992).

The Trauma History Questionnaire (THQ; Green, 1996) is a 24-item questionnaire that assesses the lifetime occurrence of a variety of traumatic events in three categories: crime, general disaster/trauma, and sexual and physical assault experiences. Participants responded "yes/no" to the specific event, the number of times the event occurred, and the age of the occurrence.

The PTSD Checklist-Civilian Version (PCL-C; Weathers, Huska, & Keane, 1991) was completed by participants. The PCL-C was developed to assess PTSD symptoms among civilian (i.e., non combat) populations. The measure has 17 items, each corresponding to a specific DSM-IV PTSD symptom. Participants responded to how much they have been bothered by each symptom in the past month, using a 5-point Likert scale that ranged from "not at all" (1) to "extremely (5). The scale had strong internal consistency (alpha = .90), which is consistent with research among other chronically ill patients (Andrykowski & Cordova, 1998).

Drug and Alcohol Use Survey (Koopman, Rosario, & Rotheram-Borus, 1994; Rotheram-Borus, Koopman, & Bradley, 1988) was used to assess recent (i.e., last three months) use of alcohol, marijuana/hashish, cocaine/crack, hallucinogens, barbiturates, over-the-counter medication, heroin, amphetamines and prescription medication.

The Center for Epidemiological Studies Depression Scale (CES-D; Radloff, 1977) was used to assess depression. It is a 20-item inventory that measures depressive symptoms over the previous week and is scored on a 4-point Likert scale indicating the frequency of symptoms. Scores can range from 0 to 60. The mean score for the general population is approximately 8. Scores of 15 or below indicate low depressive symptoms, scores between 16 and 22 indicate probable depression, and scores of 23 or higher indicate significant depression (Radloff & Locke, 1986). The measure demonstrated strong internal consistency (alpha = .90).

The Sexual Risk Behavior Assessment Schedule (Meyer-Bahlburg, Ehrhardt, Exner, & Gruen, 1988) assessed lifetime and current (last three months) sexual activity. Sexual activities with male and female partners occurring in the past three months were assessed using an adapted version of this instrument. We defined unprotected sexual activity is defined in this paper as any penile-vaginal and anal sexual intercourse in which a condom was not used.

RESULTS

Consistent with our previous research (Gore-Felton et al., 2001), a significant proportion of the sample had experienced trauma such that over half (58%) reported at least one traumatic experience severe enough to meet criterion A1 definition for PTSD disorder. Almost a quarter of the sample (22%) reported moderate to severe trauma symptoms (i.e., total PCL-C greater than or equal to 50), suggesting a likely association with a formal PTSD diagnosis. The frequency of reported trauma symptoms in this sample is not surprising given the range and frequency of different types of traumatic experiences (see Table 1). One-third (33%) of the sample reported unprotected sexual intercourse with a wide range in the reported number of times that unprotected sex occurred within the past 3 months (0 to 112; see Table 1).

Almost half of the sample (48%) reported being in a situation where they might be killed; similarly, 48% reported seeing someone killed. It is important to note that no one reported ever being in combat. Fifty percent reported seeing a non-funeral dead body and 49% reported being forced to have sex by a stranger. Being attacked with a weapon was experienced by 46% of the sample, while 28% reported being attacked without a weapon. Being beaten was endorsed by 25% of the sample, while 69% stated someone had tried to rob them.

On average the sample reported moderate amounts of depression (M = 18.0, SD = 12.0, range = 0-48). More than one-third of the sample (36%) reported scores of 23 or higher, indicating significant depression. Overall depression scores were significantly associated with overall trauma symptoms on the PCL-C ($r = .61$, $p < .0001$). We did not find significant associations between substance use in the past three months

TABLE 1. Descriptive Statistics of Trauma Severity, Trauma-Related Symptoms, and Unprotected Sex

Variable	Mean	SD	Range
Crime-related trauma (# times)	6.8	15.5	0-107
Sexual coercion trauma (# times)	6.4	22.1	0-151
Physical abuse trauma (# times)	3.3	7.2	0-30
PCL-C (total score)	37.8	14.0	17-73
Unprotected sex past 3 months (# times)	5.8	20.7	0-112

and trauma symptoms. However, we did find positive associations between severity of sexual abuse and alcohol use ($r = .26, p < .03$) as well as hallucinogen use ($r = .29$ $p < .03$) during the past three months.

An examination of trauma symptoms and risk behavior showed moderate to severe trauma symptoms were significantly correlated with unprotected sexual intercourse during the past three months ($r = .38, p < .03$). In particular, greater symptoms of intrusion and avoidance were associated with unprotected sex ($r = .29, p < .05$ and $r = .35, p < .02$, respectively). Moreover, reliving the traumatic event (i.e., experiencing flashbacks, having nightmares) was significantly and positively associated with having more partners in the past 3 months ($r = .36, p < .05$). As expected, multiple traumas were positively associated with greater overall trauma scores ($M = 43$, $SD = 14$, range 17-79, $r = .86, p < .0001$). Reliving the trauma, avoiding stimulus that reminds individual of traumatic event, and hyperarousal symptoms were each significantly and positively associated with depression ($r = .46, p < .01$; $r = .66, p < .001$; $r = .64, p < .001$, respectively).

We conducted a hierarchical multiple regression analysis using unprotected vaginal and/or anal intercourse as the dependent variable. Because the risk variable was positively skewed (J-shaped) we used logarithmic transformation on this variable so that it would approach a normal distribution and therefore appropriate for regression analysis (Cohen, 1988). To examine the influence of demographic variables on sexual risk, we first entered age, gender, ethnicity, and education using stepwise procedure. In the next block, we entered alcohol, hallucinogen, amphetamine, heroin, crack, and cocaine use in the past three months using stepwise procedure. In the third and final block, we entered severity of interpersonal crime, physical coercion and sexual coercion from the THQ, and the three classical symptom clusters of PTSD (i.e., intrusion, avoidance, and arousal) from the PCL-C instrument using stepwise procedure. We retained only those variables that were significant into the final model (Table 2). Being male, greater severity of sexual coercion, greater symptoms of intrusion, and less symptoms of avoidance were positively associated with greater sexual risk behavior (i.e., unprotected sex) in the past three months, [$F(4, 56) = 9.66$, adj$R^2 = .46$, $p < .0001$)].

DISCUSSION

Consistent with previous research, the results of this study suggest that there is a substantial amount of trauma (Kimerling et al., 1999,

TABLE 2. Multiple Regression Model Predicting Unprotected Sex in Past Three Months

Independent variable	Beta	SE	T
Male gender	.25	6.95	2.00*
Severity sexual coercion	.46	.10	3.89**
Avoidance symptoms	−.50	2.22	3.91**
Intrusion symptoms	.47	2.57	3.50**

*p = .05.
**p < .001.

Zierler et al., 2000) and trauma-related symptoms (Kimerling et al., 1999; Gore-Felton et al., 2001) among HIV-positive adults. Adding to the growing body of literature illustrating a link between trauma and HIV risk (Allers & Benjack, 1991; Allers et al., 1993; Carballo-Diéguez & Dolezal, 1995; Kalichman et al., 2001), we also found a positive relationship between trauma experience and sexual risk behavior. Indeed, in our sample, individuals that reported greater severity of sexual coercion (i.e., the number times the coercion occurred) were more likely to report more unprotected sex during the past three months. This is important because it's not simply the experience of sexual coercion that is related to sexual risk behavior, but it appears that the severity of abuse is an important correlate of sexual risk behavior. This is consistent with our finding that greater trauma-related symptoms were associated with risk behavior such that individuals that experienced greater intrusion symptoms (e.g., nightmares) were more likely to report unprotected sex during the past three months. Avoidant symptoms were associated with sexual risk behavior in that individuals reporting greater symptoms of avoidance were less likely to report unprotected sexual intercourse in the past three months. A possible explanation for this may be that individuals who suffer from avoidant symptoms may also experience greater disruption in their ability to establish or maintain intimate relationships resulting in decreased opportunities to engage in risky sexual behavior. To our knowledge, this is the first study that found that trauma-related symptoms can influence sexual risk behavior and, just as important, that not all trauma-related symptoms influence sexual behavior in the same manner.

Previous cross-sectional studies have shown that sexual abuse is the event that most often leads to posttraumatic stress disorder (PTSD) among women (Breslau et al., 1991; Resnick, Kilpatrick, Dansky, Saunders, & Best, 1993). This coupled with evidence that there is a risk of increased drug disorders that is associated with an increased risk for HIV among individuals with PTSD has led some researchers to hypothesize that PTSD psychopathology may mediate the relationship between abuse and sexual risk behavior (Miller, 1999). This study provides preliminary support for this hypothesis that merits further investigation. Specifically, we found that severity of sexual coercion and intrusive trauma symptoms were positively associated with unprotected sexual intercourse. Because of the cross-sectional design of this study we were unable to determine the mediating effects on sexual coercion and sexual risk behavior. It may be that individuals who suffer multiple sexual coercion episodes over time are not able to recognize situations that may lead to coercion or lack the skills required to communicate or negotiate safer sexual behavior with their sexual partners. Similarly, greater intrusive symptoms may impede one's ability to establish relationships where it is safe to discuss using condoms without the threat of violence, particularly among individuals that have a history of being in sexually coercive relationships.

The interpretation of this study's results needs to done in consideration of the methodological limitations. First, the self-report measures may introduce reporting error or bias into the data. Second, the cross-sectional design of the study precludes the possibility of establishing the direction of causality between the variables that were examined. Therefore, it is possible that the factors of gender, severity of sexual coercion, intrusion, and avoidance that were associated with sexual risk behavior may, indeed, influence sexual risk behavior, or be affected by sexual risk behavior, or be related to a third, unknown variable or set of variables not included in this study. Third, the small sample size limits our ability to detect significance because the regression coefficients are less stable than they would be with a larger sample size. Moreover, the generalizability of these findings can only be made to persons living with HIV/AIDS because we did not include a comparison group of healthy individuals or individuals with other medical diagnoses.

Given the study limitations, it is important to note that we were able to account for almost 50% of the variance in sexual risk behavior by examining trauma experiences and trauma-related symptoms among a diverse sample of HIV-positive adults. This suggests a robust relationship between traumatic life experiences, psychopathology and sexual risk behavior among HIV-positive adults. Moreover, the finding that the severity of sexual coercion experiences is associated with sexual risk behavior underscores the urgent need to understand the mechanisms that mediate and or moderate this relationship.

Indeed, as medical interventions continue to improve health and increase the overall life expectancies of people living with HIV/AIDS there will be more people living with HIV, suggesting HIV prevention efforts need to broaden their focus to include HIV-positive populations. Incorporating the assessment of trauma and the treatment of trauma-related symptoms among HIV-positive men and women may be a particularly effective method of reducing sexual risk behavior. Thus, intervention and prevention efforts may be able to thwart new infections by developing strategies that not only build skills needed to prevent HIV but effectively target psychological symptoms and behaviors which occur within the context of traumatic life experiences.

Understanding factors associated with HIV risk is critical to developing interventions that will effectively reduce HIV infection rates, particularly among populations where the epidemic is rising. Future research needs to examine the association between trauma experiences and symptoms to sexual risk behavior among larger samples of HIV-positive individuals as well as among populations that are HIV negative using longitudinal designs to determine cause and effect.

REFERENCES

Allers, C.T., & Benjack, K.J. (1991). Connections between childhood abuse and HIV infection. *Journal of Counseling & Development*, *70*, 309-313.

Allers, C.T., Benjack, K.J., White, J., & Rousey, J. T. (1993). HIV vulnerability and the adult survivor of childhood sexual abuse. *Child Abuse & Neglect*, *17*, 291-298.

Andrykowski, M.A., & Cordova, M.J. (1998). Factors associated with PTSD symptoms following treatment for breast cancer: test of the Andersen model. *Journal of Traumatic Stress*, *11*, 189-203.

Axelrod, J., Myers, H.F., Durvasula, R.S., Wyatt, G.E., & Cheng M. (1999). The impact of relationship violence, HIV, and ethnicity on adjustment in women. *Cultural Diversity & Ethic Minority Psychology*, *5*, 263-275.

Breslau, N., Davis, G.C., Andreski, P., & Peterson, E. (1991). Traumatic events and posttraumatic stress disorder in an urban population of young adults. *Archives of General Psychiatry*, *48*, 216-222.

Brown, G.R., & Rundell, J.R. (1990). Prospective study of psychiatric morbidity in HIV-seropositive women without AIDS. *General Hospital Psychiatry*, *12*, 30-35.

Catañia, J., Coates, T., Kegeles, S., Fullilove, M.T, Peterson, J., Marin, B., Siegel, S., & Hulley, S. (1992). Condom use in multi-ethnic neighborhoods of San Francisco: The population-based AMEN (AIDS in multiethnic neighborhoods) study. *American Journal of Public Health*, *82*, 284-287.

Carballo-Diéguez, A., & Dolezal, C. (1995). Association between history of childhood sexual abuse and adult HIV-risk sexual behavior in Puerto Rican men who have sex with men. *Child Abuse & Neglect, 19*, 595-605.

Centers for Disease Control and Prevention (1992). 1993 revised classification system for HIV infection expanded surveillance case definition for AIDS among adolescents and adults. *Morbidity and Mortality Weekly Report, 41*, 1-15.

Centers for Disease Control and Prevention (1994). *HIV/AIDS surveillance report, vol. 6(1).* Atlanta, GA: Author.

Centers for Disease Control and Prevention (1996). *HIV/AIDS surveillance report, vol. 8(2).* Atlanta, GA: Author.

Centers for Disease Control and Prevention (1999). *HIV/AIDS surveillance report, vol. 11(1).* Atlanta, GA: Author.

Cohen, J. (1988). *Statistical power analysis for the behavioral sciences (2nd ed.).* New Jersey: Lawrence Erlbaum Associates.

Des Jarlais, D.C., & Friedman, S.R. (1988). The psychology of preventing AIDS among intravenous drug users. *American Psychologist, 43*, 865-870.

Des Jarlais, D.C., Friedman, S.R., & Casriel, C. (1990). Target groups for preventing AIDS among intravenous drug users: The "Hard" data studies. *Journal of Consulting and Clinical Psychology, 58*, 50-56.

Fullilove, M.T., Fullilove, R.E., Smith, M., Michael, C., Panzer, P.G., & Wallace, R. (1993). Violence, trauma, and post-traumatic stress disorder among women drug users. *Journal of Traumatic Stress, 6*, 533-543.

Gore-Felton, C., Butler, L.D., & Koopman, C. (2001). HIV disease, violence, and posttraumatic stress. *Focus, 16*(6), 5-6.

Gore-Felton, C., Brondino, M., Benotsch, E., Kalichman, S., & Cage, M. (in submission). Trauma symptoms, sexual behaviors, and substance abuse: Correlates of childhood trauma and HIV risk behavior among gay and bisexual men.

Green, B.L. (1996). Psychometric review of Trauma History Questionnaire (Self-Report). In B.H. Stamm (Ed.). *Measurement of stress, trauma, and adaptation* (pp. 366-369). Lutherville, MD: Sidran Press.

He, H., McCoy, H.V., Stevens, S.J., & Stark, M.J. (1998). Violence and HIV sexual risk among female sex partners of male drug users. *Women & Health, 27* (1-2), 161-175.

Hearst N., & Hulley, S.B. (1988). Preventing the heterosexual spread of AIDS: Are we giving our patients the best advice? *JAMA, 259*, 2428-2432.

Holmes, S.A. (1998). AIDS deaths in U.S. drop by nearly half as infections go on. *New York Times*, October 8, p. A1.

Joint United Nations Programme on HIV/AIDS/World Health Organization (1998). *The global epidemic.* Geneva, Switzerland: Author.

Kalichman, S.C. (2000). HIV transmission risk behaviors of men and women living with HIV/AIDS: Prevalence, predictors, and emerging clinical interventions. *Clinical Psychology: Science and Practice, 7*(1), 32-47.

Kalichman, S.C., Benotsch, E., Rompa, D., Gore-Felton, C., Austin, J., Webster, L., DiFonzo, K., Buckles, J., Kyomugrsha, F., & Simpson, D. (2001). Unwanted sexual experiences and sexual risks among gay and bisexual men: Associations among revictimization, substance use and psychiatric symptoms. *The Journal of Sex Research*, *38*(1), 1-9.

Keane, T.M., & Wolfe, J. (1990). Comorbidity in post-traumatic stress disorder: An analysis of community and clinical studies. *Journal of Applied Social Psychology*, *50*, 138-140.

Kimerling, R., Calhoun, K.S., Forehand, R., Armistead, L., Morse, E., Morse, P., Clark, R., & Clark, L. (1999). Traumatic stress in HIV-infected women. *AIDS Education and Prevention*, *11*, 321-330.

Klein, S.J., & Birkhead, G.S. (2000). Domestic violence and HIV/AIDS, Letter to the Editor. *American Journal of Public Health*, *90*, 1648.

Koopman, C., Rosario, M., & Rotheram-Borus, M.J. (1994). Runaways' drug and alcohol use and its relationship to sexual risk behavior. *Addictive Behaviors*, *19*, 95-103.

Kulka, R.A., Schlenger, W.E., Fairbank, J.A., Hough, R.L., Jordan, B.K., & Marmar, C.R. (1990). *Trauma and the vietnam war generation: Report of findings from the national vietnam veterans' readjustment study*. New York: Brunner/Mazel.

Lemp, G.F., Hirozawa, A.M., Givertz, D., Nieri, G.N., Anderson, L., Lindegren, M.L., Janssen, R.S., & Katz, M.D. (1994). Seroprevalence of HIV and risk behaviors among young homosexual and bisexual men: The San Francisco/Berkeley young men's survey. *JAMA*, *272*, 449-454.

Letellier, P. (1996). Twin epidemics: Domestic violence and HIV infection among gay and bisexual men. In C.M. Renzetti, & C.H. Miley (Eds.), *Violence in gay and lesbian domestic partnerships* (pp. 69-81). New York: The Haworth Press, Inc.

Martin, J.A., Smith, B.L., Mathews, T.J., & Ventura, S.J. (1999). Births and deaths: preliminary data for 1998. *National Vital Statistics Reports*, *47*(25), 1-8.

Meyer-Bahlburg, H.F., Ehrhardt, A.A., Exner, T.M., & Gruen, R.S. (1988). *Sexual Risk Behavior Assessment Schedule–Youth*. New York: New York State Psychiatric Institute and Department of Psychiatry, College of Physicians and Surgeons, Columbia University.

Miller, M. (1999). A model to explain the relationship between sexual abuse and HIV risk among women. *AIDS Care*, *11*(1), 3-20.

Ostrow, D.G., VanRaden, M.J., Fox, R., Kingsley, L.A. Dudley, J. & Kaslow, R,A. (1990). Recreational drug use and sexual behavior change in a cohort of homosexual men: The multicenter AIDS cohort study (MACS). *AIDS*, *4*, 759-765.

Penkower, K., Dew, M.A., Kingsley, L., Becker, J.T., Satz, P., Schaerf, F.W., & Sheridan, K. (1991). Behavioral, health and psychosocial factors and risk for HIV infection among sexually active homosexual men: the multicenter AIDS cohort study. *American Journal of Public Health*, *81*, 194-196.

Radloff, L.S. (1977). The CES-D Scale: A new self-report depression scale for research in the general population. *Applied Psychological Measurement*, *1*, 385-401.

Radloff, L.S., & Locke, B.Z. (1986). The community mental health assessment survey and CES-D scale. In M. Weissman, J. Myers, & C. Ross (Eds.), *Community surveys of psychiatric disorders* (pp. 177-187). New Brunswick, NJ: Rutgers University Press.

Resnick, H.S., Kilpatrick, D.G., Dansky, B.S., Saunders, B.E., & Best, C.L. (1993). Prevalence of civilian trauma and posttraumatic stress disorder in a representative national sample of women. *Journal of Consulting & Clinical Psychology, 61*, 984-991.

Rotheram-Borus, M.J., Koopman, C., & Bradley, J.S. (1988). *Drug and alcohol use survey for adolescents*. New York: Division of Child Psychiatry, Department of Psychiatry, College of Physicians and Surgeons, Columbia University.

Stall, R., Ekstrand, M., Pollack, L., McKusick, L., & Coates T.J. (1990). Relapse from safer sex: The next challenge for AIDS prevention efforts. *Journal of Acquired Immune Deficiency Syndromes, 3*, 1181-1187.

Strunin, L., & Hingson, R. (1992). Alcohol, drugs, and adolescent sexual behavior. *International Journal of the Addictions, 27*(2), 129-146.

U.S. Census Bureau. (1999). *Resident population estimates of the United States by sex, race, and Hispanic origin: April 1, 1990 to November 1, 1999*. Washington, DC: Author.

Weathers, F.W., Huska, J.A., & Keane, T.M. (1991). *The PTSD checklist-civilian version (PCL-C)*. (Available from F.W. Weathers, National Center for PTSD, Boston Veterans Affairs Medical Center, 150 S. Huntington Avenue, Boston, MA 02130).

Weiss, D.S., Marmar, C.R., Schlenger, W.E., Fairbank, J.A., Jordan, B.K., Houugh, R.L., & Kulka, R.A.. (1992). The prevalence of lifetime and partial post-traumatic stress disorder in Vietnam theater veterans. *Journal of Traumatic Stress, 5*, 365-376.

Zierler, S., Cunningham, W.E., Anderson, R., Shapiro, M.F., Bozzette, S.A., Nakazono, T., Morton, S., Crystal, S., Stein, M., Turner, B., & St. Clair, P. (2000). Violence victimization after HIV infection in a US probability sample of adult patients in primary care. *American Journal of Public Health, 90*, 208-215.

Sexual Orientation Conflict in the Dissociative Disorders

Colin A. Ross, MD

I have been running a hospital-based Trauma Program for nine years. During this time period there have been approximately three thousand admissions to the Program. Almost all of these individuals meet diagnostic criteria for either dissociative identity disorder or dissociative disorder not otherwise specified. Although I have never done a formal tabulation, 90%-95% of the people admitted to the Program are women, which is consistent with all large series of dissociative disorder cases (Putnam, Guroff, Silberman, Barban, & Post, 1986; Ross, Norton & Wozney, 1989; Ross, Miller, Reagor, Bjornson, Fraser, & Anderson, 1990).

Colin A. Ross is affiliated with The Colin A. Ross Institute for Psychological Trauma, 1701 Gateway, Suite 349, Richardson, TX 75080 (E-mail: rossinst@rossinst.com).

[Haworth co-indexing entry note]: "Sexual Orientation Conflict in the Dissociative Disorders." Ross, Colin A. Co-published simultaneously in *Journal of Trauma & Dissociation* (The Haworth Medical Press, an imprint of The Haworth Press, Inc.) Vol. 3, No. 4, 2002, pp. 137-146; and: *Trauma and Sexuality: The Effects of Childhood Sexual, Physical, and Emotional Abuse on Sexuality Identity and Behavior* (ed: James A. Chu, and Elizabeth S. Bowman) The Haworth Medical Press, an imprint of The Haworth Press, Inc., 2002, pp. 137-146. Single or multiple copies of this article are available for a fee from The Haworth Document Delivery Service [1-800-HAWORTH, 9:00 a.m. - 5:00 p.m. (EST). E-mail address: getinfo@haworthpressinc.com].

Likewise, although I have never done a formal survey, I have observed that a high percentage of individuals admitted to the Program are primarily or exclusively homosexual in their current sexual orientation. This is true of both the men and the women. Since only about 4% of the general population is homosexual (Green, 1980), it is clear that some kind of sampling bias is taking place. The sampling bias is a scientific and logical problem; its causes are unknown and there is no relevant body of thought in the dissociative disorders literature, other than the work of Margo Rivera (1996).

The purpose of this opinion piece is to provide some preliminary discussion of the problem, and to call for more research and thought about it. Based on my own clinical experience and discussion with colleagues, it appears that similar high rates of homosexuality are characteristic of most or all specialty inpatient programs treating dissociative disorders.

In order to provide some preliminary information, I surveyed 34 patients in my Trauma Program during the weeks of February 12 and March 5, 2001 concerning their sexual orientation. Patients were asked to complete a brief questionnaire asking about gender, age, current diagnoses, and sexual behavior in adulthood. Diagnoses inquired about were dissociative identity disorder (DID), dissociative disorder not otherwise specified (DDNOS) and posttraumatic stress disorder (PTSD). Possible responses to sexual orientation were exclusively heterosexual, mostly heterosexual, bisexual, mostly homosexual, and exclusively homosexual. The questionnaire directed the respondents to report their "sexual behavior" not their thoughts, feelings or attitudes.

Five men and twenty-nine women completed the questionnaire. The men had an average age of 40.8 years with a range of 25-48 years. Of the men, one reported a diagnosis of DID, three reported DDNOS and three reported PTSD. Three were exclusively heterosexual and two (40%) were bisexual.

The twenty-nine women had an average age of 37.3 years, with a range of 20-52 years. Seventeen responded that they had DID, 6 DDNOS, and 8 PTSD. Nineteen women said they were exclusively heterosexual, three mostly heterosexual, two bisexual, three mostly homosexual, one said she was asexual and one did not respond. Thus, of the women, 17.2% said that they were bisexual or mostly homosexual.

The very informal and preliminary survey data suggest that the percentage of Trauma Program patients who are bisexual or homosexual is far higher than the base rate in the general population.

ASSUMPTIONS AND LOGICAL POSSIBILITIES

The scientific problem is: Why are the rates of homosexuality so high among inpatients with dissociative disorders? In thinking about the problem, I make the following assumptions:

- Moral and religious controversies about homosexuality are not relevant to the problem
- The problem is logical and scientific
- Trauma Program patients are a highly biased sample, therefore any conclusions drawn from this population have limited generalizability
- Scientifically, the relative weights of genetic and environmental causation of homosexuality are unknown
- The trauma relevant to the sampling bias problem includes physical, sexual, emotional and verbal abuse, neglect, violence, family chaos and loss of primary caretakers–it is not limited to sexual abuse

I will consider two logical possibilities concerning the sampling bias:

- The high rate of homosexuality is driven by trauma
- Most of these individuals would have been bisexual or primarily homosexual even if not traumatized

If one assumes that the high rate of homosexuality in the Trauma Program is trauma-driven, then a number of observations and predictions follow logically. Assuming that the homosexuality is trauma-driven does not require an assumption that it is pathological. Becoming predominantly homosexual in response to abuse and neglect by opposite-gender family members could be simply an understandable, normal human reaction. Similarly, "paranoia" can be a normal response to real political persecution, in which case it is not a symptom of mental disorder.

LOGICAL PROBLEMS ARISING FROM THE ASSUMPTION THAT THE HOMOSEXUALITY IS PREDOMINANTLY TRAUMA-DRIVEN

Since 90%-95% of the Trauma Program clientele are women, and since almost all of them have been abused and/or neglected by male family members, it is not hard to understand why they would turn to women for emotional and sexual intimacy–men are too destructive and frightening. However, a logical problem arises immediately, because many of the patients have also been extensively abused and neglected by female first-degree relatives. If one assumes that male perpetrators push the women in the direction of homosexuality, then one should assume that female offenders push them in the direction of heterosexuality. One is then at a loss to explain the net outcome of these two counter-balancing forces.

Another problem arises. Although the sample of men in the Trauma Program is much smaller, their rate of homosexuality appears equal to or higher than the women's, and it is still an order of magnitude above the base rate in the general population. Following the logic of the trauma analysis, one would have to assume that female perpetrators had more influence than male perpetrators in the men's families, and this influence would have to be far out of proportion to reasonable assumptions.

LOGICAL PROBLEMS ARISING FROM THE ASSUMPTION THAT MANY TRAUMA PROGRAM PATIENTS WOULD HAVE BEEN HOMOSEXUAL EVEN IF NOT TRAUMATIZED

If one assumes an endogenous and fixed homosexual orientation at birth, then why are such a high proportion Trauma Program clientele homosexual? The Program is not defined as a gay and lesbian program. There is no body of theory in the field stating that clientele should be predominantly homosexual. In fact, except for Rivera (1996), the problem of trauma and sexual orientation has not been discussed in the dissociative disorders field. Rivera assumes that sexual orientation is determined by biology, choice and social factors in a mix that varies from one individual to the next. Her analysis is consistent with the trauma model solution to the sampling bias problem in the Trauma Program.

As an alternative hypothesis, one could propose that persons born homosexual are more prone to formation of dissociative disorders, which would explain why a relatively high percentage of the patients in the Program are homosexual. Conflict over sexual orientation could then become a fifth etiological pathway to dissociative identity disorder and dissociative disorder, not otherwise specified (Ross, 1997). In our culture, institutionalized homophobia controls social attitudes in a punitive fashion. Whichever assumption we make about the inborn versus acquired nature of homosexuality, in our society, the gay child is taught to hate him or herself. This hatred of self may even drive a fundamental dissociation between the sexual identity and the executive self, which may then become heterosexual in reaction formation.

In this model, severe chronic trauma can be sufficient to cause DID or DDNOS in a heterosexual child. However, the trauma dose must be set relatively high for this to occur, except in individuals with very low thresholds for formation of a dissociative disorder. For the 4% of individuals who are either born or become homosexual, in contrast, the trauma dose required for formation of a dissociative disorder could be lower because of society's punitive attitude towards homosexuality. The homosexual child automatically experiences trauma simply by being homosexual and may even experience dissociation between the executive self and the sexual self. The additional trauma required to reach the diagnostic threshold is therefore less than that required by the heterosexual child. Thus, the homosexual child subjected to chronic trauma may be particularly prone to develop a dissociative disorder.

We seem to have arrived at a solution of the sampling bias problem. Unfortunately, we have not because the magnitude of the effect is too great. We are jumping from a base rate of 4% to a rate as high as 40% in the Trauma Program. This cannot be explained by a model of heightened susceptibility of homosexual children to develop dissociative disorders. This model would have to be the major etiological pathway to chronic, complex dissociative disorders, at least among inpatients in specialty programs. Such a conclusion could be accepted only with a major shift of thinking in the field. The role of other forms of trauma would have to be drastically reduced. In addition, other changes in our clinical thinking would follow logically.

CLINICAL HYPOTHESES THAT FOLLOW FROM GENDER IDENTITY CONFLICTS AND SEXUAL ABUSE

About two-thirds of dissociative identity disorder patients have opposite gender alter personalities (Putnam et al., 1986; Ross et al., 1989). This is not at all surprising. Using the example of a girl with an endogenous heterosexual orientation who is sexually abused by her father, it is easy to understand the formation of several types of alter personality. Male personalities may be formed as tough protectors or as male sexual offenders through identification with the aggressor. Heterosexual male offender personalities may sexually victimize women in order to shift from the victim to the perpetrator position, and in order to undo the childhood trauma.

Non-offender male heterosexual alter personalities provide a device for healthier sexual intimacy with women while avoiding the fear and conflict linked to the identity of female incest victim. The heterosexual male alter personality in a female body also provides a defense against conflict concerning lesbian sexual behavior. Such alter personalities are based on trauma-driven reaction formation to the primary heterosexual identity.

Homosexual male alter personalities permit sexual intimacy with men, while dissociating the fear and conflict linked to the identity of female incest victim. In this instance, the reaction formation is to the trauma-driven fear and phobia, rather than to the endogenous sexual orientation.

In women, heterosexual female alter personalities may work as heterosexual prostitutes in order to be in the perpetrator/controller position and in an effort to undo childhood sexual victimization by men. Or, homosexual female alter personalities may sexually victimize women in order to be in the perpetrator position while avoiding the phobic fear of sexual contact with men. In a healthier adaptation, lesbian alter personalities may experience adult sexual intimacy with women in reaction formation to the endogenous sexual orientation and in phobic avoidance of men.

These permutations and combinations illustrate a core point of Margo Rivera's (1996) thesis: the relative health and maturity of an alter personality's sexual behavior depends only to a minor degree on whether the partner is of the same or opposite gender. The same physical behavior can have opposite motivations, be relatively healthy or pathological, and be ego-syntonic or dystonic to the host personality, depending on the nature of the alter personality in executive control at the time, and the array of defenses on which it is founded.

If this observation is generalized to the population as a whole, we arrive at Rivera's thesis that sexual orientation is determined by a mix of biology, environment and choice in most or all people. Consider the situation of the child born lesbian who is sexually abused by her father. She will gravitate strongly to an ego-syntonic lesbian adaptation for two reasons; her endogenous orientation and her trauma experience. She will develop alter personalities that have sex with men only in reaction formation to her orientation and her trauma experience. Post-integration she will have a healthy homosexual orientation.

But what if the lesbian child is sexually abused by her mother? What if the gay boy is sexually abused by his father? In these situations, we would expect different patterns of alter personalities and defenses. The gay boy sexually abused by male relatives is at higher risk for formation of female heterosexual prostitute alter personalities than male heterosexual prostitute alter personalities because of a drive to be in the perpetrator/controller position with respect to male sexual partners. He is also at higher risk to develop female lesbian personalities to avoid identification with his abusive male father. Reaction formation to his homosexuality in this child would also drive the formation of male heterosexual personalities.

Since all permutations and combinations of alter personality gender identity, sexual orientation and defense are possible, research predictions about the frequencies of types of alter personality in different scenarios are pointless. All outcomes of the data could be accounted for and none could be refuted, simply by varying the permutations. However, understanding the dynamics should be relevant in psychotherapy.

Some psychotherapy clients do not achieve normal sexual arousal and orgasm even though the client is in the late pre-integration phase of therapy. One might make two assumptions about such a client if she is a woman: that her endogenous sexual orientation is heterosexual; and that the deepest impact of paternal incest and ambivalent attachment to the perpetrator have not yet been resolved. However, in some cases, perhaps, the fundamental problem is actually her own internalized homophobia. Perhaps the deepest conflict, dissociation and self-hatred are due to endogenous lesbianism, in a subgroup of such cases. The best efforts of the client to attain a normal heterosexual adjustment are doomed to failure, in this scenario, as is conventional trauma therapy for paternal incest.

Internalized homophobia could also be a driver for memories of paternal incest in lesbian women who explain their sexual aversion to men by a trauma myth, in order to avoid dealing with and resolving their self-hatred, which is in fact based on internalized punitive attitudes to their endogenous homosexuality. A history of paternal incest is more acceptable in some social groups than is lesbianism, and it provides the benefits of the victim role.

Why are there no fathers in our culture claiming that therapists have implanted false memories of homosexual paternal incest? Perhaps men do not create myths of paternal incest because the stigma of paternal incest against boys is too high and because paternal incest leads to suspicions of endogenous homosexuality in the victim for boys more than it does for girls.

Finally, if one assumes that the rates of endogenous homosexuality are the same in boys and girls, and further assumes that the rates of trauma are the same in heterosexual and homosexual children, overall, then why are 90% -95% of trauma Program patients women? Conventional explanations cite the differential effects of trauma on boys and girls and the tendency for men to avoid seeking help. However, another explanation would have to be a greater stigma attached to male than female homosexuality in our culture. Men would be more driven to avoid trauma therapy because they are more driven to suppress and avoid their recognition of their own homosexuality.

The purpose of these thoughts and speculations is to stimulate further research and discussion. I have observed the sampling bias in sexual orientation among hospital-based Trauma Program patients over a period of nine years. Whatever the exact prevalence of predominant and/or exclusive homosexual orientation among the clientele, it is clearly an order of magnitude greater than the base rate in the general population. The dissociative disorders field has no satisfactory model to explain the sampling bias, and the problem has received virtually no consideration in the literature.

RESEARCH QUESTIONS AND STRATEGIES

Scientifically, the challenge is to transform clinical hunches and ideas into testable hypotheses. It is the data derived from tests of hypotheses that are relevant, not one's ideological position on an issue or problem. Ideology may be a source of scientific hypotheses, but these must be tested, otherwise there is disagreement and political warfare, but no science.

We lack even the most basic data relevant to the sampling bias problem. First, we need systematic data about the rates of different forms of chronic childhood trauma in heterosexual and homosexual adults. Simultaneously, we need basic data on the rates of homosexuality in trauma populations. There should be a minimum of five categories in such research: exclusively and predominantly heterosexual, bisexual, and predominantly and exclusively homosexual. We need systematic data on the genders of primary perpetrators in the families of these five categories, and we need it for the full range of different types of trauma.

Once such preliminary data are gathered, where to next? This is where we hit a dead end. There is no body of theory in the dissociative disorders field that leads to a set of testable scientific hypotheses. What would be the goal of such research? Would it be to investigate the nature-nurture controversy about the causes of homosexuality? Would it be to improve our treatment models? As a field, do we require guidelines for professional policy and treatment strategies concerning homosexuality? Should the sampling bias problem be addressed in the Treatment Guidelines of the International Society for the Study of Dissociation?

I have formulated the questions, but I don't have the answers. I do know for sure that there is a large sampling bias problem. I know for sure that it has not been addressed in the dissociative disorders literature. And I know that silence is not a reasonable position to take, at either the general literature or the International Society for the Study of Dissociation levels.

The next step, it seems to me, should be discussion in the *Journal of Trauma and Dissociation*, at annual meetings and in the Newsletter of the International Society for the Study of Dissociation. The Society's members have a wealth of relevant experience because of their extensive work with many different types of alter personalities. There is no better demonstration of the plasticity and countless permutations and combinations of defense inherent in various sexual orientations, crossed gender identities and sexual behaviors than the pantheon of alter personalities in dissociative identity disorder. Nor does any other condition demonstrate so clearly that the gender of sexual partner is only one of many factors to be considered in making a clinical judgment about the psychological health of a sexual behavior.

I am not aware of a demonstrated sampling bias in sexual orientation for any other Axis I or II diagnostic category or treatment population. Again, however, we lack even the most basic information about rates of homosexuality in different clinical samples. I predict that the percentage of a given clinical population that is homosexual correlates strongly with the average number of Axis I and II disorders lifetime, and with the total trauma dose, however that is measured.

REFERENCES

Green, R. (1980). Homosexuality. In H.I. Kaplan, A.M. Freedman, & B.J. Sadock (Eds.), *Comprehensive textbook of psychiatry, Vol. III* (pp. 1763-1770). Baltimore: Williams & Wilkins.

Putnam, F.W., Guroff, J.J., Silberman, E.K., Barban, L., & Post, R.M. (1986). The clinical phenomenology of multiple personality disorder: Review of 100 recent cases. *Journal of Clinical Psychiatry, 47*, 285-293.

Rivera, M. (1996). *More alike than different: Treating severe dissociative trauma survivors*. Toronto: University of Toronto Press.

Ross, C.A. (1997). *Dissociative identity disorder: Diagnosis, clinical features, and treatment of multiple personality*. New York: John Wiley & Sons.

Ross, C.A., Miller, S.D., Bjornson, L., Fraser, G.A., & Anderson, G. (1990). Structured interview data on 102 cases of multiple personality disorder from four centers. *American Journal of Psychiatry, 147*, 596-601.

Ross, C.A., Norton, G.R., & Wozney, K. (1989). Multiple personality disorder: An analysis of 236 cases. *Canadian Journal of Psychiatry, 34*, 413-418.

Index